Medical Leadership:
From the Dark Side to Centre Stage

Medical Leadership: From the Dark Side to Centre Stage

PETER SPURGEON

Director, Institute for Clinical Leadership
Medical School, University of Warwick

JOHN CLARK

Senior Fellow, The King's Fund
(Formerly, Director of Medical Leadership,
NHS Institute for Innovation and Improvement)

and

CHRIS HAM

Chief Executive, The King's Fund

Foreword by
Sir Bruce Keogh

NHS Medical Director

Radcliffe Publishing
London • New York

Radcliffe Publishing Ltd
33–41 Dallington Street
London
EC1V 0BB
United Kingdom

www.radcliffepublishing.com

Electronic catalogue and worldwide online ordering facility.

British Library Cataloguing in Publication Data

A catalogue record for this book is available from the British Library.

ISBN-13: 978 184619 246 3

The paper used for the text pages of this book is FSC certified. FSC (The Forest Stewardship Council) is an international network to promote responsible management of the world's forests.

Typeset by KnowledgeWorks Global Ltd, Chennai, India
Printed and bound by TJI Digital, Padstow, Cornwall, UK

Contents

Foreword

The future direction of healthcare around the world will be determined by a mix of national economics, public and professional expectations and global technology. Sometimes these interests will be in conflict, particularly as governments increasingly focus on the economic impact of societal demands and technological growth on healthcare delivery systems. These considerations are likely to accelerate in the aftermath of the recent global financial crisis. Never before has the quality of leadership in healthcare been more important.

The quality of leadership and management defines the difference between excellence and mediocrity and success and failure for all organisations. In my view, good leaders inspire others and are able to align them towards a common goal through a clear vision. Good managers, on the other hand, simplify and streamline the way organisations work to achieve their goals and maximise potential. These are two quite different functions. Not all leaders are good managers, but most effective managers are also good leaders; the two sets of qualities are complementary to effective organisation performance.

In healthcare provider organisations the quality of clinical leadership always underpins the difference between exceptional and adequate or pedestrian clinical services which in aggregate determine the overall effectiveness, safety and reputation of every healthcare organisation. Similarly, effective clinical leadership in commissioning organisations brings perspective and challenge which in turn drives up clinical quality for the whole health economy. So good clinical leadership is not an end in itself, it is a means to achieving high-performing healthcare systems.

Young doctors are inspired by good clinicians who are intellectually adept, who bring forensic scrutiny to their diagnostic and therapeutic routines, who are kind to their patients and who exhibit a comprehensive mixture of compassion and professionalism. Such doctors may have no managerial inclination, yet they are highly influential and essential leaders if our NHS is to flourish.

Doctors also seek leadership from medical royal colleges and specialist associations with whom they identify on matters of clinical quality, standards of care and training of the next generation. Therefore, clinical leadership across the NHS may take many forms ranging from frontline leaders who provide excellent service, through a spectrum of clinical innovators and academics, to those who provide professional leadership through their professional bodies or through managerial involvement at various levels in their employing institution.

Successful medical leaders are usually, but not always, experienced and credible clinicians with good people skills, who look beyond the boundaries of their own specialty or institution, who are positive and perseverant and who are prepared to take reasonable risks to achieve their goals. Most importantly they know how to engage their colleagues and effect change. They understand the principles of organisational performance and the balance between professional autonomy and corporate behaviour.

The problem is that over the years we have paid too little attention to developing clinical leadership and management skills in a coherent fashion either in undergraduate or postgraduate education. This has led to an expansion of highly qualified, non-clinical, professional healthcare managers to administer an increasingly complex NHS. Inevitably the two groups of professionals will have differing perspectives, which are addressed in Chapter 2. It seems to me that there is an enormous amount to be gained by training systems that maximise the synergy between the two professional groups, and this can be facilitated by the comprehensive application of the Medical Leadership Competency Framework across the NHS.

This book examines the historical context of how the UK NHS arrived at its current position in terms of the involvement of doctors in the wider organisational context. Lessons are drawn from comparison with systems overseas. Some exciting and critical developments are described in this text, not least the embedding of the Medical Leadership Competency Framework as a statutory element of the training and development of all doctors, evidence of the link between enhanced medical engagement and organisational performance and finally the establishment of a new Faculty of Medical Leadership and Management. The last development is a culmination of a major national project 'Enhancing Engagement in Medical Leadership' led by two of the authors (Spurgeon and Clark). The new Faculty can provide continuity from the existing project work and also give impetus to taking forward further developments in this vital sphere.

The text is a comprehensive account of the key aspects of medical leadership, but it is also readable and accessible. I can thoroughly recommend it as a read for junior and senior doctors, non-clinical and clinical managers and those taking on formal leadership roles.

Professor Sir Bruce Keogh
NHS Medical Director
April 2011

List of figures

List of tables

List of boxes

CHAPTER 1

An introduction to medical leadership and a perspective on this text

'Clinicians are expected to offer leadership and, where they have the appropriate skills, take senior leadership and management posts in research, education and service delivery. Formal leadership positions will be at a variety of levels from within the clinical team, to service lines, to departments, to organisations and ultimately the whole NHS. It requires a new obligation to step up, work with other leaders, both clinical and managerial, and change the system where this would benefit patients' (Darzi, 2008).

The motivation for this book on medical leadership was partially triggered by Lord Darzi's review of the health system culminating in the publication of *High Quality Care for All* in 2008. Policy analysts in the future may well see his strong messages about the importance of getting clinicians, and particularly doctors, more engaged in leading service improvements as a defining moment in the way in which health services in the United Kingdom are organised and led.

As the book was being finalised the new coalition government in the UK was consulting on its reform agenda for the NHS (England). Whilst much of the detail had yet to be resolved, it is very clear that the movement towards medical engagement and leadership promulgated latterly by Lord Darzi and others was to be strongly reinforced particularly through the emerging GP commissioning consortia.

The aim of this chapter is to introduce the topic of medical leadership and also to offer an overview of the key issues that are explored in more depth in subsequent chapters.

This movement did not start with the strong emphasis given to medical leadership by the Darzi Report. Doctors have been involved in the running of health services, locally, nationally and internationally, since the pioneers who initiated and organised health services many centuries ago. What is new is the emerging evidence of the relationship between the extent to which doctors are engaged in the planning, prioritization and shaping of services and the wider performance of the organisation.

We should at the outset stress that this is a book about medical leadership and engagement. Too often, commentators use the term 'clinical leadership' when clearly meaning 'medical leadership'. We make no apology for focusing on doctors; other texts usefully cover the role the wider range of clinical professionals play in health systems. Much of the content of policy directions and statements prefer to use the term 'clinical leadership' when all the subsequent text is focused on doctors. The evidence is that major changes to the way in which healthcare is delivered are driven by doctors. They are, de facto, the major decision-makers regarding the use of resources. This is not to detract from the key role other clinical professionals and non-clinical managers and leaders play. Delivery of healthcare is a team activity with all members having a major contribution to make to improve health and the way in which services are delivered.

Much of what we have to say about doctors being more involved in management, leadership and transformation can be applied to other clinical professions, but this is not the remit of this particular book. Medical leadership is a particular focus within the NHS currently and, we anticipate, for the foreseeable future.

At the time of publication, less than 5% of chief executives in the NHS are from medical backgrounds. Whilst there are some senior policymakers who seek to increase this, we don't subscribe to this view per se. There is no evidence thus far that concludes medical chief executives are more effective than non-medical leaders. However, as Chapter 7 describes, there is evidence of the links between medical engagement and performance. Chapter 8 outlines how doctors in the future will be required to attain an agreed set of management and leadership competences at all levels of their training and careers. Our contention is that, as more doctors recognise their responsibility to the wider system of care and not just individual patients, more will want to assume leadership roles at all levels, including potentially as chief executives.

The set of leadership competences for doctors embodied in the joint NHS Institute for Innovation and Improvement and Academy of Medical Royal Colleges Medical Leadership Competency Framework can equally apply to all clinical professionals. This view is now being reviewed by the NHS National Leadership Council and likely to be accepted by all clinical professional bodies.

To better understand the current strategies around medical leadership and engagement it is important to have an appreciation of the ways in which doctors have been involved in management, leadership and transformation of services. We suggest that the journey can be summarised as a movement from major domination preceding the setting-up of the NHS in 1948 through a period of disenfranchisement thereafter until perhaps the reorganisation of the health service in 1974. We contend that by this time some doctors, generally reluctantly, accepted representative roles. The Cogwheel Reports between 1967 and 1974 have had a significant impact on the way in which hospital services have been organised, i.e. around specialties ever since. The Reports also started the process whereby doctors initially took on representative roles for their specialty Cogwheel Division to and then to assuming executive responsibility for their specialty business unit and the concept of Service Line Management increasingly being introduced in Foundation NHS Trusts in England.

This shift from representation to accountability was reinforced by the Griffiths Report published in 1983 and further endorsed by the Resource Management Initiative in 1986 and the establishment of Clinical Directorates. The Griffiths view back in the early 1980s has continued to be stressed by Darzi and many other initiatives as outlined in more detail in Chapter 5. Put simply, Griffiths could not see how a service, department or organisation could be managed effectively unless it was managed by those who commit resources.

We also explore how the profession itself has changed over the same period as the policy and organisational arrangements have moved on. Whereas management and leadership were frequently dismissed by doctors and medical leaders in derogatory terms in previous eras, the medical profession is now very positively espousing the importance of doctors assuming leadership roles at all levels of training and careers and stressing their inclusion in the definition of a good doctor.

We explore in more detail why many of the initiatives introduced over the past 60 years have perhaps only been partially successful. We suggest that both managers and doctors represent two very powerful groups. Unlike many other countries, the United Kingdom has experienced a very strong managerialist culture, particularly over the past 25 years, which has often led to major conflict between clinicians and managers.

Trying to achieve some congruence between the individualistic nature of clinical practice and professionalism and the managers' broader population and organisational perspective is an inevitable area of potential conflict and tension. The exercise of clinical autonomy is a crucial part of the application of knowledge acquired by doctors through their medical training. As Oni (1995) suggests, at worst some doctors will view managers as 'agents of government to control the expert power of the professional'.

The doctor:manager conflict is perhaps a stereotyped portrayal often reinforced by media coverage, including television dramas that delight in exaggerating the gap between the clinicians' desire to provide the highest quality and quantity of care unfettered by resource constraints against the managers' need to control expenditure within allocated budgets. This latter demand has been accentuated in recent years by the increased pressure on managers to meet government performance targets particularly over access and waiting time. It is perhaps this 'battle-zone' of the performance management philosophy inherent in the concept of managerialism that creates the real challenge for health leaders. Seeking to get some shared and balanced understandings between the individual doctor's desire to deliver high quality care to every patient and the managers' need to deliver political and organisational imperatives has been a long-standing challenge. As we explore in later chapters, the more this potential chasm can be minimised the more likely local communities will benefit from high quality and efficient services. It is not an impossible dream, but understanding the different motivations and perspectives is perhaps the critical issue. Various reports into where this chasm has led to disastrous implications for patients have consistently confirmed this dysfunctionality. There can be no greater argument or incentive for seeking to reduce the divide.

It is as Barnett *et al.* (2004) contend: there is a need for a 'convergence of cultures' and not a contest between any perceived or real emphasised differences. Finding common ground is the challenge. Who could deny that this is around service improvement and patient safety? Throughout this book we shall keep coming back to this need to find alignment of values and aspirations.

In Chapter 4 we describe the recent trends in healthcare reform and their implications for medical leadership. All too frequently health reforms leave us with a reality gap, i.e. the difference between the stated desired outcomes and improvements of reform and the reality. We postulate there have been four major phases of health reform in the NHS since the late 1970s, i.e.:

Phase 1	Late 1970s/early 1980s	Cost containment at the macro level
Phase 2	Late 1980s/early 1990s	Micro efficiency and responsiveness to users
Phase 3	Late 1990s	Rationing and priority-setting
Phase 4	Current	Improving quality and safety of care

Whilst these four phases broadly apply to all four home countries, the approach to implementation and the governance arrangements to support the initiatives have differed particularly since the introduction of devolved governments at the end of the 20th century.

We widen the analysis of reforms and draw on other European and international studies which confirm that the gap between rhetoric and reality is not peculiar to the NHS. Whilst one diagnosis is around weaknesses in policy design, we also explore the power of clinical professionals and particularly doctors to frustrate the intentions of the policy-makers.

Reflecting on the various NHS reforms of the past 30 years or so, it is evident that all have recognised the importance of involving doctors in the reforms, but it is perhaps only the recent Darzi Report that sees clinical engagement and leadership as central to health reform. Even more recently, Liberating the NHS (2010) has seen general practitioners move to centre stage in England through their central role in commissioning services.

We explore some of the factors that hinder the active engagement of doctors in leading health reforms and suggest that both policymakers and those implementing these need to understand what Henry Mintzberg described as 'professional bureaucracies' (Mintzberg, 1979). Perhaps the current drive for greater engagement of doctors in leading reforms both nationally and locally suggests that there is a better explicit understanding of this concept by both policymakers and the medical profession.

Throughout the book we provide examples of how high performing organisations are typified by strong partnerships between doctors and managers at all levels. Distributed or shared leadership is gaining prominence within new leadership paradigms of, for example, microsystems and service line management approaches.

We reflect that, whilst healthcare reform since the 1970s has highlighted the need to engage doctors more effectively in reforms, it is only perhaps over the past couple of years that there is a shared appreciation by policymakers, the medical profession and NHS leaders that the rhetoric reality gap can only be closed by a genuine commitment to greater medical engagement and leadership.

The evidence for the greater engagement of doctors is perhaps best summarised in Chapter 7 where we explore some of the inter-related concepts of performance, leadership and engagement. We draw on some of the growing body of evidence suggesting that good management practice and effective leadership can have a positive impact on organisational performance.

The authors have been involved in a major national study looking at the relationship between medical engagement and organisational performance. Much of the limited work around the impact of clinical engagement has hitherto tended to describe different models and approaches within specific organisations that appear to have led to a range of defined benefits, e.g. greater staff satisfaction and commitment, reduced staff turnover, greater patient satisfaction, etc.

In Chapter 7 we outline how an existing Professional Engagement Scale was adapted and tested to provide a discrete medical engagement focus. The Medical Engagement Scale (MES) is based around three meta levels:

Meta Scale 1   Working in an open culture
Meta Scale 2   Having purpose and direction
Meta Scale 3   Feeling valued and empowered

A detailed analysis of the comparison between the MES Index and overall Healthcare Commission (now Care Quality Commission) ratings is provided in Chapter 7, but it is apparent that organisations scoring more highly on engagement are independently assessed as superior in performance across a number of areas. In addition, more detailed statistical analyses reveal a large number of significant relationships between the medical engagement index and other independently collected performance markers, e.g. standardised mortality rates and the National Patient Safety Agency data on incidents resulting in severe harm.

The evidence from this study provides confirmatory support for the policy reform agenda based around more doctors leading improvements in quality, safety and productivity. It also supports the notion that shared and distributed leadership at all levels is more likely to produce the benefits sought. Many local studies have demonstrated the impact of effective medical engagement, but the medical engagement scale appears to offer a powerful and validated tool for organisations to benchmark themselves against other hospitals and primary care trusts and to identify areas for improvement. Lessons from those Trusts with high levels of engagement should also be useful for the new GP Commissioning Consortia as they are established.

We also draw on a study examining the ways in which doctors are involved in medical leadership in a number of countries and how they were prepared for leadership roles. Edwards, Kornacki and Silversin (2002) contend that there has been a breakdown in the implicit deal between doctors, patients, employers and society around what the parties to the relationship give and what they get in return. They describe the changing societal context within which doctors now practise, including greater accountability for their performance, need to deliver patient-centred care and to work collectively with other clinicians and staff to improve quality.

This change in the psychological compact is not an NHS or a UK phenomenon. Most countries are seeking to find ways of encouraging doctors to be more engaged in service improvements and to assume leadership roles. The evidence from research confirms that quality initiatives that fail to engage doctors tend to have a limited impact.

A number of American health organisations, e.g. Kaiser Permanente, Mayo Clinic and Geisinger, provide examples of what can be achieved through high levels of medical engagement and leadership.

From the countries reviewed in Chapter 6 it is clear that there is no system that provides THE answer. There are some countries, e.g. Japan and Turkey, where it is mandatory for a doctor to be the chief executive. However, there is no evidence that this leads to greater engagement of other doctors or indeed that it results in higher performance. What is evident is that all systems have some doctors who are better prepared for their management-leadership roles than others. Equally, all systems have great examples of service improvement initiatives and of organisations with enviable cultures of medical and staff engagement. The challenge for any health system is how to spread and adopt best practice such that it is the norm and not an isolated exemplar.

The implementation of the Medical Leadership Competency Framework (MLCF) developed by the NHS Institute for Innovation and Improvement and the Academy of Medical Royal Colleges appears to be a first internationally, and other countries are keen to adopt variants of the approach.

Given that this book is about medical leadership, it would be wrong not to provide a brief discussion of a few of the theories and approaches to leadership that are perhaps of particular relevance to this overall discussion. There are thousands of texts seeking to define leadership and the most effective styles, and this has led us to conclude that there are almost an infinite number of ways in which leadership can be exercised.

Given the context of healthcare delivery and the importance of team-working, we favour a model of shared or distributed leadership. In Chapter 8 we describe in detail the Medical Leadership Competency Framework which applies to all doctors at all levels in their practitioner roles. It is not aimed at specific positional leaders but as a set of competences that should be fully integrated into the medical role.

Essentially, shared leadership is about the quality of the interaction rather than formal positions and is evaluated by how well people work together. It is where everyone is engaged in acts of leadership, where communication and making sense of conflict ensure that the process is democratic, honest and ethical and where the common goal in healthcare of improved services to patients is based on evidence and professional judgement (*see* Chapter 3).

As we explore the links between medical engagement and organisational performance in Chapter 7, the concept of shared leadership becomes even more pertinent. Medical engagement has traditionally tended to focus on those few doctors who assume formal positional roles, e.g. clinical directors, medical directors, commissioning leads, etc. Indeed many chief executives when asked about medical engagement within their trusts immediately discuss their medical leadership organisational structure. The desire to create more inclusive cultures where doctors at all levels are actively engaged in improvement of services requires a movement away from the more hierarchical models of the past few decades and a transition to a much more distributed or shared leadership approach.

We have already referred to the development of the joint NHS Institute and Academy Medical Leadership Competency Framework (MLCF) and how this is likely to have a profound impact on the way in which doctors view their managerial and leadership responsibilities in future. Historically, there has been a tension between doctors and managers. By creating ways in which medical students and postgraduate trainee doctors recognise much earlier in their training and careers their responsibility to improve services for populations of patients as well as for their individual patients, a new form of professional bureaucracy within the NHS should emerge. The current reforms focus on seeking greater medical engagement and leadership but from within a historical culture where such change is a real challenge. The future looks more promising with young doctors being positively encouraged to develop management and leadership competences and to lead service improvement initiatives.

In Chapter 8 we explore the use of competences in medical education, training and practice but with a particular focus on those management and leadership competences that are relevant to doctors increasing their contribution to quality and productivity improvements. Historically, the medical profession has led the way in terms of innovative approaches to curricula design, learning and assessment. We examine some of these approaches across broader medical education both nationally and internationally and particularly focus on the relevance of the CanMEDS Roles Framework (Frank, 2005). This has influenced many medical professional bodies in a number of countries to rethink their definition of medical professionalism and the role of 'a good doctor'.

This Framework, along with others, influenced the development of the MLCF. The Leadership Framework is unique and has now informed the revision of *Tomorrow's Doctors* (2009) for medical students and the revision of all specialty curricula for postgraduate doctors. It is also informing revalidation standards and criteria for consultants and general practitioners.

It would be wrong to imply that some of these competences have never been incorporated previously in medical education and training. Many will have been covered under professionalism or other themes. However, the MLCF and its endorsement by all the medical professional, regulatory and educational bodies provides a nationally consistent set of standards which all medical students and doctors should attain.

The Framework is being supported by e-learning packages and advice on assessment. It provides a great opportunity to excite medical students and young doctors about the important role they can play in contributing to, and leading, service improvements. Any educational and training support must be seen to be relevant to doctors if the benefits for health systems and populations are to be realised. The focus must therefore be around service improvement and recognising the importance of developing self-awareness and impact on others as well as on working within teams.

In Chapter 9 we explore some of the practical initiatives being taken in the NHS to operationalise the MLCF and to provide new opportunities for doctors to gain managerial and leadership experiences and competences at earlier stages in their careers. We offer a number of examples of how medical students and young postgraduate doctors are being offered, and accepting, innovative options to contribute to the health improvement movement.

The explicit need for medical students and postgraduate doctors to attain competence within the MLCF has to be balanced with creating the climate where they passionately *want* to accomplish this. Any mandatory requirement will not achieve the cultural change of greater engagement by doctors in planning, delivery and transformation of services alone. What is needed is a cultural transformation or social movement that encourages doctors to be engaged and where the non-clinical leaders genuinely seek to get doctors driving reforms and to be part of the leadership team at all levels (*see* Chapter 10).

This is a critical time for the future of the medical profession. As Rosen and Dewar (2004) suggest, there are unprecedented challenges arising from the changing expectations of patients, governments and managers. They suggest that whilst doctors remain 'professionals' the traditional image of what this means in practice is changing. Throughout this book we will provide examples and reasons why this is happening – and at a pace. Rosen and Dewar provide a range of factors why society is forcing a new compact between doctors, patients and government.

It is very evident that the expectation of these stakeholders is changing. This book explores these challenges and seeks to examine the factors that have influenced a major paradigm shift. The involvement of doctors in planning, delivery and transformation of services is no longer an optional extra: it is a mission critical to the whole social movement around improving the quality of care for patients and productivity. We are embarking on a new approach to delivering healthcare with doctors very much more engaged and perhaps increasingly centre stage.

The following chapters will describe, and critically analyse, the factors leading to this new approach. Only time will tell whether the anticipated benefits will be realised.

REFERENCES

Barnett P, Malcolm L, Wright L, *et al*. Professional leadership and organisational change: progress towards developing a quality culture in New Zealand's health system. *The New Zealand Medical Journal*. 2004; **117**(1198): 1–11.

Darzi A. *High Quality Care for All: NHS next stage review final report*. London: Department of Health; 2008.

Department of Health. *Equity and excellence: liberating the NHS*. London: Department of Health; July 2010.

Edwards N, Kornacki M, Silversin J. Unhappy doctors: what are the causes and what can be done? *BMJ*. 2002; **324**; 835–8.

Frank JR, editor. *The CanMEDS Physician Competency Framework. Better standards. Better physicians. Better care*. Ottawa: The Royal College of Physicians and Surgeons of Canada; 2005.

Mintzberg H. *The Structuring of Organisations: a synthesis of the research*. Englewood Cliffs, NJ: Prentice-Hall; 1979.

Oni OO. Who should lead in the NHS? *J Manag Med*. 1995: 9(4); 31–4.

Rosen R, Dewar S. *On Being a Doctor: redefining medical professionalism for better patient care*. London: King's Fund; 2004.

West M, Borrill C, Dawson J, *et al*. The link between the management of employees and patient mortality in acute hospitals. *Int J Hum Resour Man*. 2002: **13**(8); 1299–310.

CHAPTER 2

Doctors and managers: differing perspectives

INTRODUCTION

There have been many attempts to encourage greater involvement of doctors in the management and leadership of the organisations in which they work. Despite the relatively high-profile nature of some of these initiatives with support from government and national leaders, the outcomes have not been particularly successful. This suggests that structural or mechanistic approaches are not enough and that there may be a more underlying and significant difficulty. This chapter will explore what might be an important aspect of the problem: that of the differing perspectives held by doctors and managers about the focus and functioning of the health service. The NHS is frequently described as comprising a series of 'tribes', and newcomers are often surprised, if not dismayed, by the strength and resilience of the different views held.

Degeling *et al.* (2001) have explored the views of doctors, managers, medical managers and nurses in the context of health system reform. They point to sometimes quite subtle differences in the understanding and importance attached to common issues. These differences seem to be sustained in a range of settings and may originate from training, expectations and cultures. Degeling and his colleagues, and Spurgeon and Flanagan (2000) described distinct sub-cultures within NHS organisations.

Managers and doctors represent two very powerful groups, and thereby what may be matters of emphasis become important, so much so that they may lead to conflict. The situation is not new but it persists, taking on varying manifestations as particular models of organisational arrangements are put forward.

Hunter (2005), reviewing 25 years of health policy reform, sees the cult of managerialism as an important process, whether in early attempts to impose accountability on clinicians for the resources they use (early 1970 and 1980s) through to the modernisation programme initiated and continuing in 1997. Hunter describes the equation as increased investment but attached to a requirement to adopt major changes in working practices to promote the quality of services and patient experience. The mechanisms used to implement modernisation, targets and regulation can give rise to dysfunctional behaviour in clinicians resentful at the encroachment of managers and management onto their territory, and the challenge it presents to their professionalism.

The use of the term 'territory' is instructive here as it suggests conflict, turf wars and ultimately a relationship between doctors and managers mediated through status and power. The dynamic interplay of power politics can manifest itself at many levels, individual and institutional. A recent Healthcare Commission (2009) report into the quality of care at Mid Staffordshire Hospitals NHS Foundation Trust suggested that a managerial focus upon achieving Foundation status, attaining financial balance and meeting performance targets had distracted the organisation from ensuring quality of care to patients was the priority. If concerns were raised it appears, at least from the outside, that the medical voice was overwhelmed by the managerial priority. At an individual level, too-direct interventions by individual managers in what may be perceived as the clinical domain can spark hostilities that can be long lasting and difficult to overcome. Irrespective of the level of focus of the conflict it is clear that such division is not good for patients. We look later (Chapter 5) into the history of how current conflicts may have arisen, but in order to move beyond the past we need to understand better the nature of differing perspectives.

DIFFERENT PERSPECTIVES: BASIS AND IMPLICATIONS

Numerous studies report the impact or implications of the differing perspectives, but before considering these it may be helpful to look at two particular accounts, Thorne (2001) and Plochg and Klazing (2005), who attempt to set out the theoretical underpinnings of the divergence in the views of managers and doctors. Thorne sets her argument within the framework of domains of jurisdiction particularly in the workplace. Who should control and supervise work, and who is qualified to do which parts of it? A pure and typically historic jurisdiction is defined for professional bodies by knowledge and expertise. This is generally stable and changes quite slowly. However, in a workplace setting such as the NHS there is an organisational context to these jurisdictions or boundaries. External events, like reform processes, cause disturbance and can lead to disputes between professional groups as to territory or dominance. The promotion of doctors as managers is just such a process causing managers and doctors to think about definitions of their areas. In these circumstances many are defensive and a few see the opportunities. In a different context, these few are sometimes described as 'early adopters' but can often appear isolated and rejected by the majority. Later studies will illustrate this.

Thorne takes clinical directors as the focus of her thesis, arguing that they embody the tension between managerial and professional structures. The basis of medical power/dominance can be traced to three interlocking concepts:

- Control of the labour market (Friedson, 2001)
- Expertise expressed as clinical autonomy (Starr, 1982)
- Self-regulation.

In terms of the labour market the numbers of students entering medical school have been quite tightly controlled. Only recently has this restriction on numbers been eased by increased intakes and the establishment of new medical schools. Traditionally the restriction on numbers has resulted in doctors having high incomes, high social status and public legitimacy. Having passed into the profession, Ackroyd (1996) described the process as being in a powerful clinical 'enclave'. This is seen in the relatively flat structure of the profession, with all consultants notionally having equal power and standing. This situation is in marked contrast to the hierarchical and accountable structures of management.

The dominance of the medical profession and its exercise of clinical autonomy is to a large extent based on the medicalisation of healthcare. As a consequence of this prevailing model it is only doctors who can define 'medical work', its diagnosis and treatment. This singular role creates a dependency for health organisations (Ackroyd, 1996) and enables doctors to determine priorities, ration care and commit scarce resources (Calman, 1994). Changes are emerging in this particular context, as resource pressures have led to a variety of role substitutions where other professions have taken over parts of what was previously the role of the doctor.

Nurse specialists, for example, have been a significant part of the approach to meeting the European Working Time Directive restriction on hours doctors can work (48 hours) by assuming some of the tasks of junior doctors. Again, as with increased entry to the medical profession, it is likely that the continuation of extended roles for other groups will have an impact upon the status of doctors. Initially this is likely to be quite painful (as experienced by the profession) but ultimately may free doctors to become more integrated into the managed health community – those managed *by it* and those *members of* the management process.

The exercise of clinical autonomy is a crucial part of the application of the knowledge acquired through medical training. The profession's main regulatory body, the General Medical Council (GMC), acts to preserve and prescribe the boundaries to this autonomy and freedom to exercise clinical judgement. Once more this area too is undergoing significant change, with rapidly increasing lay involvement with the GMC and also more guidelines and protocols determining the nature of care to be given to a type of patient and thus limiting individual clinical decision-making. This is a sensitive and contentious area in the doctor-manager relationship. At its worst some doctors will view managers as 'agents of government, given "structural power" to control the "expert" power of the professional' (Oni, 1995). The use of government targets and their pursuit by managers with a responsibility to achieve them has proved a major source of difficulty and conflict.

The second theoretical approach to exploring the relationship between doctors and managers comes from Plochg and Klazinga (2005) and is related to the notion of introducing clinical governance programmes. They note how many of these seem

to have failed and suggest that improvement may be made through a better understanding of the perspectives of the two groups. Drawing once more on Friedson's
(2001) concepts of professionalism, they suggest that doctors have the privilege of
dividing and co-ordinating their own work processes, resulting in various specialties and subspecialties. These domains or areas are maintained and protected by a
number of strategies:

- expertise is expanded and differentiated, so thereby only those with acknowledged competence can function in the area
- delegation of certain tasks to non-clinicians whilst keeping overall charge of
  the domain
- striving to keep their own group of patients who thus have a dependent and
  particular relationship with the specialty
- participating in specialist activities, e.g. pharmaceuticals committee and guide-
  line development.

There are real benefits (to patients) of these strategies – notably, a culture of clinical excellence whereby knowledge is continuously updated to reinforce the value
of the specialty. However, this drive for exclusiveness creates an inward orientation
and encourages an individualistic culture. Even within the profession, therefore,
there can be a disconnect from other medical colleagues, let alone from the organisational context.

In direct contrast the 'management science' perspective endeavours to devise
ways of best organising the workforce and creating procedures to ensure that the
organisation meets its goals. Within these rules and structures different staff groups
will at various times be aligned or ill-fitting, with consequent tension and disrup-
tion. This tension is particularly acute in what Mintzberg (1983) described as 'professional bureaucracies' where knowledge and expertise are at a premium in the
successful functioning of the organisation. Managers have used a range of initiatives such as guidelines, evidence-based medicine and regulation (Checkland *et al.*,
2004) to promote standardisation of processes. Whilst difficult to argue against
standardisation in the form of consistent treatment, it is an approach that is uncom-
fortable with high levels of individually based expertise. There are issues here going
far beyond this particular context of how society in attempting to demystify and
reduce the power of professions by codifying what was once discretionary decision
making may be destroying the essence of public confidence in long-standing professions and their regulatory bodies.

There are then some clear historic and underlying reasons why doctors and managers may form differing perspectives and take quite contrasting views of the same
process. Numerous health service initiatives have foundered on this divide, and
many studies have documented experiences of these processes and how they play
out at the workplace. Before discussing approaches to overcoming the problem it
may be useful to illustrate the difficulties in context.

DOCTORS AND MANAGERS: HOW THE DIVIDE IS MANIFEST

A rather straightforward statement of the problem comes from Australia, where Jorm and Kam (2004) describe doctors as having 'their own all-pervading culture' which centres on their occupational identity, its exclusiveness and a tendency towards traditional values. From this base, Jorm and Kam argue (with some evidence) that doctors are adept at diverting the goals of many improvement initiatives that do not obviously resonate with their own position. Conflict derived from a very strong cultural identity is a source of many issues, whether with individual managers or at an organisational level. Collectively there seem to be two main types of areas where this can be seen: (a) in the tension, ambiguity and discomfort stemming from doctors undertaking managerial and leadership roles, and (b) the performance management philosophy inherent in the concept of managerialism.

(a) **The doctor-manager role conflict**

McDermott *et al.* (2002) offer a study of a major reform in the Irish health system that took as a key goal the greater involvement of clinicians in management roles. Interestingly, in their conclusions they allude to the contrast in dealing with change within a medical context as opposed to outside it. 'While scientific advances constantly drive clinicians to adopt new treatments and techniques, this capacity for change does not appear to include adaptation of the doctor's role in society'. They point also to a frequently voiced concern of having to make the transition from an independent, individually based, patient-focused decision to one that is collective and corporate.

Forbes *et al.* (2004) make use of the concept of the psychological contract by which employees enter into an agreed relationship with their employer. Changes in the status of the contract will have an impact upon the motivation and behaviour of the employee. Forbes and colleagues suggest that doctors enter healthcare organisations with a set of values, assumptions and ethical premises based upon their professional culture. How they experience the organisation, often as represented by managers, will make a difference to their own commitment to the psychological contract. It was to explore this experience of management that Forbes *et al.* conducted their study using in-depth interviews with clinicians who had undertaken management roles. They identified two distinct types of doctor-manager, which they termed the 'investors' or the 'reluctants'. The former were characterised as entering management with a specific agenda which might include influencing health service delivery, or sometimes an escape from clinical pressures. Some members of this group saw themselves as natural leaders and innovators taking these skills into management as a smooth transition. A key factor in defining this group was the acceptance of management, which tended to make them proactive in developing their role and management identity. Thus they begin to acquire a new or altered identity from that with which they entered the organisation, and crucially are comfortable in the role.

In contrast, the 'reluctants' – as the name suggests – tended to enter management not because of a particular desire to do so but because they felt pressured into accepting the role. They were often quite negative about management, had had poor experience of management and hence had little commitment to the role. Such individuals were clearly lacking much satisfaction from their managerial role but equally became separated from clinical colleagues because of the role and hence suffered the worst experience of this dual position. These clinical colleagues often referred to such an individual as 'having moved to the dark side'. There is a critical thread here to the entire text in that unless the role of manager/leader becomes accepted and valued by the medical profession as a whole then the ambiguous relationship between doctors and health organisations will continue.

The cultural interplay relating to management and leadership roles has frequently focused on specific positions such as the clinical and medical director. The issues have been quite long-standing, with the difficulties seeming to continue irrespective of the particular era or initiative in question. From the outset of the 'clinical directorate' model, many authors have attempted to investigate and describe how the medical profession has responded to the desire to see them more involved in running and directing health organisations (Bruce and Hill, 1994); (Buchanan *et al.*, 1997); (Smith, 2002); (Davies and Harrison, 2003). The commonality in the accounts relates to a series of dilemmas for doctors as they interface with management roles which by their persistent presence seem to be largely unresolved.

As the studies previously mentioned have demonstrated, there is an overarching issue about the status (or lack of) attached to prescribed roles such as clinical director. Underlying this is the way management overall is perceived. Many doctors rapidly acquire a stereotypical view that management is the source of burdensome bureaucracy, that managers are antagonistic towards doctors and lack the commitment to the patient in the same way as doctors. Therefore someone choosing to go into such a role is explicitly expressing preference for another group or culture. This can in itself produce alienation from the peer group. Many doctors in formal roles of management or leadership report a sense of loss and isolation from their peers and indeed a wariness from some who project a sense of disloyalty upon them. The strength of the medical community is almost palpable in these circumstances. A linked issue that emanates from the same source is that of retaining clinical credibility if one moves from full-time clinical practice. This is an extremely powerful concept and seems peculiar to doctors even in comparison with other sectors. In most industries professional competence is assessed at entry and assumed to grow with practice; however, this experience then seems to stand one in good stead should management be the preferred career route. In medicine this does not appear to be the case. There is an established view that even after 20 years or more of practice, this cannot confer credibility if at any point direct clinical

contact is dropped. The NHS is probably on the cusp of confronting this position as more medical directors become full-time appointments. If these posts
are successful and sought after, it may be that the acceptance of doctors in other
roles (without continuing medical practice) will increase.

It is because of this credibility issue that the time allocated to medical
management within a job role has been such a significant dilemma. There
is no uniformity about how much time is appropriate for a role such as the
clinical director – typically varying from two sessions to half time. Virtually
all part-time appointees report great pressure on time and a consequent sense
of overload, perhaps also giving rise to a feeling of not being able to do the
job properly.

Key principles of medical professionalism, clinical freedom and autonomy, are seen by many to be in conflict with the collective ethos of management. At an individual clinician level there may well be moral and ethical
conflicts. However, a wider construct here is how far by responding to the call
to become more involved in the management process the profession is also
acknowledging that it too is part of the managed community of healthcare
(Spurgeon, 2001).

Finally, within the realm of role pressures it is fair to recognise the potential challenge to the individual of moving from recognised status and success
in medical practice to the uncertainty that a management role represents. The
majority of doctors make this transition with limited training for the role.
Some would argue the training that they have had (in the more scientific aspects of medicine) provides a particular difficulty to accepting the less precise,
more interpersonally dependent outcomes attached to the managerial role.
It has to date been quite unclear how the decision to accept a management
role affects career prospects. There is no career structure for such roles. Merit
awards do not appear to value contribution to management in the same way
as they do teaching and research. There has therefore been no financial incentive to become involved.

(b)   **Doctors and performance management**
As discussed above there are many influences of occupational socialisation
that create differing perspectives on the value of management to doctors as
opposed to managers. This is exacerbated or heightened by the introduction
of the more specific concept of performance management, a fundamental
component of the management process that exists at least in part to manage, contribute to or affect the performance of the organisation. Without this
notion management shrinks to that of administration which is supportive
of the organisation but has less direct influence over it. Chapter 5 explores
the continuum of moving from administration to management, and it is no
coincidence that many senior doctors hanker for the days when administrators worked to support the professionally led processes and did not challenge
them. Performance management of the organisation of course involves the

performance of individuals and hence the potential for conflict around the legitimacy of any challenge to clinical autonomy.

The same sensitivity to performance management may be seen in the way in which the appraisal system was introduced to the medical profession. In the face of a number of high-profile medical failures, the statutory and regulatory bodies could not resist the introduction of appraisal in terms of public confidence in the profession. However, in practice there was great emphasis given to the developmental focus of the appraisal process. It was recognised that this was probably the most effective way of getting appraisal established within the profession. The more confrontational assessment component of appraisal by which areas of deficiency might be identified was largely resisted. Where attempts were made to introduce such an element it was controversial and often undermined by attacking (not unreasonably) the quality of the data upon which an assessment might be based. Even for appraisal system purists who argue that it should be about the future and development opportunities, the lack of a proper performance management system and consequent absence of appropriate data illustrates how alien the concept is in the medical world.

The scientific aspects of medical training and the professions' broad endorsement of evidence-based medicine makes it somewhat surprising that an effective performance management culture has not been established. Improvement methodologies, with some notable exceptions, have been relatively slow to gain acceptance in the profession. Improvement would require clear performance standards for each task and constant monitoring to measure improvement achieved. The imposition of external performance standards and targets has been much resisted by the medical world as not relating to appropriate clinical priorities. There is undoubtedly some substance to this point, but the real issue is why so many changes had to be imposed rather than emanating from within the profession. The reason is probably to be found within the concept of clinical autonomy and the implicit model of competence within it. The exercise of professional judgement is essential to professional work across the board, but it is heavily emphasised in medicine, with GPs and consultants by dint of *being* GPs and consultants assumed to be competent. If everyone is competent there would (historically) be no need for explicit standards and measurement, because everyone would be doing the right thing. But is everyone doing the right things to the same level? Do we know and how would we know? The relatively recent emergence of patient safety as a priority does suggest levels of variability in performance standards across medical practice. Many doctors are responding to this challenge with more explicit standards, measures and improvement targets developing across a wide range of procedures.

The real point of the discussion though is to illustrate how difficult it has been for managers to enter the debate about performance even when they wanted to do so. Greener (2005) suggests that managers felt inhibited about raising individual performance standards, concerned that it might provoke more generalised resistance from a profession liable to close ranks if under threat. Until quite recently, only the strongest and most confident of managers have felt it was legitimate to challenge clinical practice. This is gradually changing with better data being available more widely and with more doctors participating in the management process and feeling it an appropriate part of the role to assess performance of colleagues. Ultimately though it will require the medical profession to more widely recognise and accept that it is part of an integrated management system and that it does not sit slightly outside it.

Reconciling different perspectives

The chapter has made clear that by training and practice managers and doctors often have different perspectives on a range of issues. The future enhanced involvement of doctors in the management process does require some reconciliation or coalescence of views so that both groups can work collaboratively and productively for the benefit of patients.

There is a need for a 'convergence of cultures' (Barnett *et al.*, 2004) and as this term suggests not a dominance or sense of one prevailing over the other. It may well be that appealing to the notion of service improvement and patient safety is something around which all groups can unite. The NHS Confederation (2003) has attempted to address the issue quite explicitly by promoting more shared training and development between managers and doctors. They call for more shared dialogue and engagement so that the different perspectives can be made explicit but can also be acknowledged and accepted as the basis for a positive partnership. Remaining chapters in this book will explore further how these premises have been taken forward.

REFERENCES

Ackroyd S. Organisation contra organisations: professions and organisational change in the United Kingdom. *Organisation Studies.* 1996; **17**(4): 599–621.

Barnett P, Malcolm L, Wright L, *et al.* Professional leadership and organisational change: progress towards developing a quality culture in New Zealand's health system. *The New Zealand Medical Journal.* 2004; **117**(1198): 1–11.

Bruce A, Hill S. Relationship between doctors and managers: the Scottish experience. *Journal of Management in Medicine.* 1994; **8**(5): 49–57.

Buchanan D, Jordan S, Preston D, *et al.* Doctors in the process. the engagement of clinical directors in hospital management. *Journal of Management in Medicine.* 1997; **11**(3): 132–50.

Calman K. The profession of medicine. *BMJ.* 1994; **309**: 1140–3.

Checkland K, Marshall M, Harrison S. Re-thinking accountability: trust versus confidence in medical practice. *Qual Saf Health Care.* 2004; **13**(2): 9–14.

Davies HTO, Harrison S. Trends in doctor-manager relationships. *BMJ.* 2003; **326**: 646–9.

Degeling P, Kennedy J, Hill M. Mediating the cultural boundaries between medicine, nursing and management – the central challenge in hospital reform. *Health Serv Manage Res.* 2001; **14**(1): 36–48.

Forbes T, Hallier J, Calder L. Doctors as managers; investors and reluctants in a dual role. *Health Serv Manage Res.* 2004; **17**(3): 1–10.

Friedson E. *The Third Logic.* Cambridge: Policy Press/Blackwell; 2001.

Greener I. health management as strategic behaviour. *Public Management Review.* 2005; **7**(1): 95–110.

Healthcare Commission (2009). *Investigation into Mid Staffordshire NHS Foundation Trust.* Available at: www.cqc.org.uk/_db/_documents/Investigation_into_Mid_Staffordshire_ NHS_Foundation_Trust.pdf (accessed 19 April 2011).

Hunter DJ. The National Health Service 1980–2005. *Public Money and Management.* 2005; 209–12.

Jorm C, Kam P. Does medical culture limit doctors' adoption of quality improvement? Lessons from Camelot. *J Health Services Research Policy.* 2004; **9**(4): 248–51.

McDermott R, Callanan I, Buttimer A. Involving Irish clinicians in hospital management roles – towards a functional integration model. *Clinician in Management.* 2002; **11**(1): 37–46.

Mintzberg H. *Structures in Fives: designing effective organisations.* Englewood Cliffs, NJ: Prentice-Hall; 1983.

Oni OO. Who should lead in the NHS? *Journal of Management in Medicine.* 1995; **9**(4): 31–4.

Plochg T, Klazinga NS. Talking towards excellence: a theoretical underpinning of the dialogue between doctors and managers. *Clinical Governance: an international journal.* 2005; **10**(1): 1–7.

Smith D. Management and medicine: strange bedfellows or partners in crime? *Clinician in Management.* 2002; **11**(4): 159–62.

Spurgeon P, Flanagan H. *Managerial Effectiveness.* Milton Keynes: Open University; 2000.

Spurgeon P. Involving clinicians in management: a challenge of perspective. *Health Care and Informatics Online.* 2001. Available at: www.hinz.org.nz/journal/2001/08/ Involving-Clinicians-in-Management-A-Challenge-of-Perspective/546 (accessed 27 May 2011).

Starr P. *The Social Transformation of American Medicine.* New York, NY: Basic Books; 1982.

The NHS Confederation Medicine and Management. *Improving Relations between Doctors and Managers.* London: NHS Confederation; 2003.

Thorne ML. Colonizing the new world of NHS management: the shifting power of professionals. *Health Serv Manage Res.* 2002; **15**: 14–26.

CHAPTER 3

Roles and models of leadership

INTRODUCTION

Many of the commentators arguing the case for enhanced medical leadership have considerable expertise in the shaping and delivery of health services at a strategic and operational level, though oddly enough, the majority do not have particular academic expertise in the study of the concept of leadership itself. As a consequence, many advocates write about leadership as if there is a single concept to which everyone adheres or alternatively without specifying any particular approach or model of leadership.

Does this rather non-specific approach to the concept of leadership matter? Probably not too much at the most general level where there is consensus as to the need for greater positive involvement of doctors in the running and development of the organisations in which they work. However, we will *see* in Chapter 7 – with regard to the concept of engagement – that when seeking to link particular behaviours or to develop leadership it does become rather more important to understand and to differentiate some of the many approaches to leadership. It is not appropriate in this chapter or indeed this text to explore over a century of leadership research, but it may be helpful to discuss one or two key aspects and to see how these might relate to the possible roles of medical leaders and how doctors might be prepared for such roles. For a full discussion of approaches to leadership the reader is referred to Northouse (2010).

LEADERSHIP – THE CONCEPT

How we talk about leadership and the language used to describe it often suggest an implicit model or concept of leadership. As Spurgeon (2007) suggests, there is a tendency to confuse the question 'who are leaders?' with 'what do leaders do?'. The former approach emphasises the notion of leadership as a personal capacity and has tended to produce an unending series of lists of personal qualities that an individual, designated as a leader, might possess. Inevitably, a paragon matching up to all these qualities does not exist. The lists seem to imply some kind of ideal type whereas the reality is that an individual may possess some of these personal characteristics to some degree. How much of each is needed to be a leader is never specified. As people do function as leaders it follows that there is an almost infinite set of combinations of personal characteristics that can enable someone to be a leader and the critical conclusion that follows is that there are lots of different ways in which leadership can be exercised.

Understanding that there is no single universal set of characteristics that define a leader goes a long way to explaining why the term leadership and all the qualities associated with it can create confusion. Also, more constructively it suggests that many individuals can contribute as leaders, but in quite different ways, depending upon their own particular set of strengths and weaknesses.

Grint (2001) suggests that the term leadership is so 'multifaceted' and that so many constructions exist that many authors in writing about leadership do not really define exactly what they mean. To a large extent this is exactly the case in the context of medical leadership.

One of the most commonly accepted definitions of leadership comes from Northouse (2010, p. 3), a major author in the field who offers 'a process whereby an individual influences a group of individuals to achieve a common goal'. The research process in leadership work has as a consequence largely centred on identifying just what is the source of influence enacted by the individual in the exercise of leadership.

Willcocks (2005) provides a very succinct account of the main approaches to understanding leadership and importantly attempts to relate these models in terms of their applicability to the medical world. The approaches he describes are grouped under the heading of:

- trait theory
- leadership styles
- contingency theory
- transactional/transformational leadership
- shared or distributed leadership.

There is a temporal sequence to the relative standing of each of these approaches, starting with trait models dominating until the 1930s. Although each model has acquired a certain dominance at a particular period in time the previous model has not entirely disappeared. The strands of thinking in one approach tend to re-emerge or linger and become encompassed in subsequent approaches, often re-framed.

TRAIT THEORY

This was the earliest of the approaches and placed great emphasis upon personal characteristics possessed by eminent leaders, usually military or political leaders. Despite a great deal of research, a rather limited set of characteristics – intelligence, self-confidence, drive, integrity and achievement – have emerged. These are hardly surprising as a list and seem almost a semantic restatement of the term leadership itself. Higgs (2003) has suggested adding emotional intelligence to the list.

In order to be of practical value the characteristics emerging as relating to leadership would need to be stable across a variety of situations and consensus exist as to the items in the list. Unfortunately, neither position holds. The trait approach also implicitly sees leadership as an innate set of qualities possessed by some and not others, therefore negating many of the attempts to train or develop such qualities.

More recently, Alimo-Metcalfe and Alban-Metcalfe (2001) have revived interest in key characteristics and how they might enable leadership. The descriptors are more sophisticated (inspirational, integrity, genuine concern, approachable) and more accommodating of a modern context, but they remain nonetheless a list and all the caveats remain – is this the only and agreed list, does a leader need all or some and how much of each, and do they apply equally in all circumstances?

The trait approach might be argued to have some resonance with the medical profession, given the emphasis placed on key personal characteristics in the selection process. But as Willcocks (2005) points out, whilst many doctors have many qualities of leadership, not all doctors possess the same qualities. There may be a different distribution in different specialties and moreover, the doctor may employ personal qualities in a primarily patient-doctor context and not necessarily in the dynamic group context of leadership.

LEADERSHIP STYLES

The style approach is in part a reaction to the deficiencies of the trait approach and its failure to recognise the impact of the situation in which leadership occurred. It is essentially a dichotomised model where leaders either focus on the task or the people involved. In reality it may be a little more blurred than this, and the notion of a choice of a style of leadership founders a little on the failure to determine whether there is a 'best' style or how one determines which style is appropriate at any one time. This same deficiency is apparent in the context of medicine, where it may be quite uncertain as to whether different specialities or groups of specialties demand particular personal characteristics.

Contingency approach

Again in a consequential development to the previously described model, this approach tries to recognise and describe the complexity of the different situations in such a way as to suggest which style may be most appropriate. Whilst an attractive model in trying to integrate style and context, it has been criticised for taking a rather narrowly defined set of situations, and as Darmer (2000) suggests it rather depends on who defines the situation in question. The approach also demands an awareness of different models of leadership and the not inconsiderable dual skills of being able to recognise when a particular approach is required, i.e. to be able to recognise the demands of the situation, and also to be able to enact whatever model seems appropriate.

In practice, in a healthcare setting experience suggests it is unlikely that there will exist a sufficiently wide selection of potential clinical leaders to be able to match style and context, or indeed that the context will be sufficiently amenable to adaptation should the designated leader seek to alter it. One can see here an explanation for many of the clashes between a clinical director and other clinical colleagues who either do not see the context in the same way as the leader or are unwilling to change it.

TRANSACTIONAL/TRANSFORMATIONAL APPROACH

This more recent strand of thinking about leadership derives in part from processes of globalisation provoking greater instability and turbulence in external environments. In these circumstances, being able to cope with constant change, to motivate and inspire others to see beyond the initial dislocation of change forces is seen as key, and this is the defining feature of transformational leadership. It is defined in contrast to the more traditional management focus (described as transactional) which seeks to establish order and control, and is perhaps better attuned to more stable external environments. This notion of transformational leadership has proved quite attractive as it projects leaders tackling unpredictable, dynamic circumstances as opposed to the more staid, steady image of the manager. However, transformational leadership is in danger of slipping back towards the trait approach, being rather elusive to measure and appearing to emphasise the charismatic, heroic (and hence rare) nature of leadership in difficult circumstances.

There is often a desire in some to see management and leadership as quite distinct, frequently raising the question: 'But are you talking about management or leadership?' Spurgeon and Cragg (2007, p. 98) argue that this is rather a false dichotomy, seeing them as more of a dimension and having a complementary relationship. They suggest that 'delivering and maintaining change inspired by leaders requires management expertise. Thus the two functions support and complement one another. They vary in emphasis and are more or less appropriate at different times depending on circumstances. Both roles are needed but it is clear that some managers will be able to offer leadership in addition, whilst some cannot. Equally many outstanding leaders are also very competent managers – but that is not necessarily the case for all leaders'.

Grint (2002) takes a rather wry look at the issue, noting that politicians will typically blame the ills of the NHS on managers for their lack of control and on leaders for failing to give direction. If nothing else it is a convenient displacement of blame. Grint raises the fascinating question of what do leaders actually do? In exploring this he describes the relationship between leaders and followers as crucial. The latter must actually assent to what the leader prescribes or the leader becomes powerless. The notion that there is a perfect leader who will get all the decisions correct or a perfectly managed system that will allow no errors is rather fanciful. The 50 years of leadership development programmes would surely have got this all sorted by now if we could invest this perfect expertise in one individual. It is more likely, as Grint suggests, that we recognise leadership as functioning at many levels throughout the organisation and that encouraging all to persuade and influence others to the appropriate action is the way leadership will actually be effective. This is very much the philosophy behind the emergence of the Medical Leadership Competency Framework (MLCF), described later in this text, since it sees the acquisition of basic competence in leadership skills by all doctors as a common and universal part of training and development as the way in which more effective leadership will be located in health systems (and to other professional groups as the MLCF is extended to these other groups).

In considering the applicability of transformational leadership to the healthcare context, there is some appeal in seeing how medical leaders with this approach might create a mood for change in their clinical colleagues. However, a tension remains in that the origin of the advocated change often seems to arise from external sources and as a consequence may be viewed with suspicion by many (especially clinicians) working within the system. Transformational leadership to be successful seems to require a true commitment and passion for the goals of the change. This may not always align well when it seems that many externally inspired changes seek to direct and control the operation of previously autonomous groups.

A more recent articulation of this issue, i.e. whether leaders really believe in what they are saying and doing, is in the concept of 'authentic leadership' (Northouse, 2010). As the name implies, such leaders are described as genuine, acting with conviction and very much representing their own personal values in what they do. This is a relatively new model of leadership, and whilst it has the appeal of a moral basis for leadership behaviour it remains unclear just how values are translated into action, and of course wars have also been fought around a leader's moral conviction. Clearly we do not all see the moral basis of actions in the same way.

These then are the main historical approaches both to the study and application of leadership. There are surely others that could be discussed as subtle departures from and adaptations of these main models. It is probably important to consider just one or two more, most notably shared leadership and adaptive leadership, as they are particularly relevant to the context of healthcare – one in particular which underpins the approach of the Medical Leadership Competency Framework, described and advocated in this text.

SHARED LEADERSHIP

Shared leadership is a more modern conception of leadership that departs from the traditional charismatic or hierarchical models. Increasingly complex problems and organisations have seen growing reliance on multidisciplinary teams. Shared leadership is an approach that can support and underpin this way of working. Shared leadership can be defined as a dynamic, interactive, influencing process among individuals in groups, with the objective to lead one another to the achievement of group or organisational goals. A key distinction between shared and traditional models of leadership is that the influence process involves more than just downward influence on subordinates by a positional leader. Leadership is distributed amongst a set of individuals instead of being centralised in the hands of a single individual who acts in the role of leader (Pearce and Conger, 2003). Each team member's individual experience, knowledge and capacity is valued and is used by the team to distribute or share the job of leadership through the team in response to each context and challenge being faced.

The multidisciplinary team has become the fastest growing organisational unit. It is no longer possible for one person or one discipline to have all of the knowledge and experience to solve the complexity of today's problems. For example, governments, in trying to find a solution to global warming, need to ensure that scientists, engineers, geographers, meteorologists, biologists, botanists, oceanographers, doctors, computer programmers, ecologists and manufacturers all bring their unique knowledge and experience to this complex problem. The breakthroughs are more likely to come from the interaction between all the differing disciplines rather than a single discipline working by itself.

This approach is equally relevant within a clinical setting. Clinicians are becoming more and more specialized as a direct result of breakthroughs in technology and science that enhance our medical knowledge. For example, for patients with cancer, teams from different specialties and with different areas of expertise, e.g. surgeons, oncologists, anaesthetists, palliative care specialists, specialist nurses, general nurses, alternative therapists, radiologists, Macmillan nurses, general practitioners, physiotherapists and others all have a contribution to make to the planning and delivery of care. Within a shared leadership model, leadership passes from individual to individual along the patient's pathway of care. This provides continuity of care for the patient through a key or caseworker without compromising standards of care. Supporting this clinical team are further networks including support services, laboratory services, manufacturers, administrators and managers.

Pearce *et al.* (2009) provide a series of examples of shared leadership success across a range of sectors. Konu and Viitanen (2008) also suggest in the Finnish health system that they saw shared leadership result in increased innovation, motivation and readiness for development. In healthcare, a shared leadership model would see the patient's care at any one point in his or her journey led by the person most able, with the key expertise to undertake the task. Shared leadership is about the quality of the interaction rather than an individual's formal position. The potential of the MLCF usage in the training of doctors to develop better communication, team working and innovation is a key reason the model is so important to the whole initiative.

HOW DOES SHARED LEADERSHIP UNDERPIN THE MLCF?

The MLCF is built on the concept of shared leadership where leadership is not restricted to people who hold designated leadership roles, and where there is a shared sense of responsibility for the success of the organisation and its services. Acts of leadership can come from anyone in the organisation, as appropriate at different times, and are focused on the achievement of the group rather than of an individual. Therefore, shared leadership actively supports effective teamwork.

In the complex world of healthcare, the belief that a single person is the leader or manager is far from reality. Leadership is a competency-based behaviour that has to come from everyone involved in healthcare. Doctors work in multidisciplinary teams focused on the needs and safety of the patient where leadership becomes the responsibility of the team. Whilst there is a formal leader of the team who is account-able for the performance of the team, the responsibility for identifying problems, solving them and implementing the appropriate action is shared by the team. The formal leader's role is to create the climate in which the team can flourish through team building, resolving conflicts and being clear about the vision. Evidence shows that shared leadership can increase risk taking, innovation and commitment, which should result in improved care for the patient and an organisation that is responsive, flexible and successful. The team members can demonstrate acts of leadership by challenging the team whilst the team establishes the norms and protocols in which the team works, managing differences by using all of the skills, knowledge and pro-fessional judgment of individual members for the benefit of the whole team.

HOW DOES SHARED LEADERSHIP RELATE TO POSITIONAL LEADERSHIP AND SELF-LEADERSHIP?

Positional leadership

Positional leadership roles are those that individuals take on within the formal structure of their organisation. Individuals are appointed to those roles on the basis of their past experience and their future potential to be part of the formal account-ability structure within an organisation. The roles themselves have a set of expecta-tions around them regardless of the individuals who occupy them. Examples of positional leadership roles within healthcare are ward managers, matrons, clini-cal directors, medical directors, nursing directors, finance directors, directors, chief executives, non-executive directors and chairmen. We understand in principle the responsibilities of these roles and would have little difficulty placing them in a for-mal diagram of the organisational hierarchy.

Shared leadership is a product of the culture of the organisation. Where an organisation is knowledge dominated and involves teams of individuals who col-lectively work towards a shared goal (such as the NHS), then shared leadership will flourish. Where the cultural norm is for hierarchy with power and influence coming from the top, then a more positional leader/follower norm will tend to exist.

In some ways healthcare has led the way, incorporating more and more individuals into multidisciplinary teams for the care of patients. Children with special needs have complex care packages that rely on the knowledge and skills of a very varied team that crosses the boundaries between healthcare, social care and education. For a child with cerebral palsy this may include specialist teachers, a special educational needs co-coordinator (SENCO), physiotherapists, occupational therapists, an audiologist, an optometrist, a community paediatrician, a hospital-based general paediatrician, a paediatric surgeon, a neurologist, community and hospital nursing teams, respite carers, social workers and others. Different events will influence and change the key issues for the child and his or her family, so the main focus of care will need move accordingly. A shared leadership approach is the model that best supports this.

The MLCF provides a helpful means to integrate shared leadership in practice. For example, if the team providing care for children with complex needs was asked to review its current service by the positional leader (in this instance the clinical director), they might start by setting out the direction of the service; they would then look at ways they could improve the service through their experience of managing the service. They would examine how they worked as a team and the personal qualities of all the team members. No individual could hold the knowledge and experience to incorporate all the dimensions, so they would use shared leadership to incorporate all the team members' views and use the interrelationship to innovate new solutions.

Hartley and Benington (2010) have recently looked at leadership specifically in the context of healthcare. It is interesting to note from their analysis of changes in healthcare provision why they see an increased demand for new and better healthcare leadership. Changing patterns of disease with greater emphasis upon prevention, lifestyle changes, community-based interventions and a more educated, demanding public will require a more outward facing form of leadership response. Similarly they suggest that the need for greater team-working in the way care is delivered, the pace of innovation and change and the demand for continuous service improvement, especially with respect to patient safety, will place tremendous demands on professional leaders working in healthcare environments.

Self-Leadership

Self-leadership is at the heart of shared leadership. Leaders need to be effective self-leaders understanding themselves and their impact on others through self-regulation, self-management and self-control. To be self-aware is to ask: 'What impact am I having?', 'Who is better at this than me?' and 'This is not working, what do I need to change?'. Self-leaders need to learn to lead themselves before they can lead others in the team or organisation (Houghton, Neck, Manz, 2002, p. 126–32). Self-leadership and shared leadership are complementary. and self-leaders will willingly and enthusiastically accept shared leadership roles and responsibilities, as this may be the only way to get the job done in complex organisations.

The MLCF recognizes that self-leadership is a building block for leadership, and this is articulated within the domain of Demonstrating Personal Qualities (*see* Chapter 8).

The MLCF also recognizes within its domain of Working with Others that, whilst some doctors will take on positional leadership roles, all doctors will, as individuals, be leaders through working with others in multidisciplinary teams, making decisions about patient care, as well as being members of organisational teams making decisions about resources, people and strategy.

ADAPTIVE LEADERSHIP

This model described by Heifetz (1994) may resonate with those struggling with apparently intractable problems in the NHS, and also with the debate surrounding management and leadership. Heifetz suggests that there is a distinction to be made between largely technical problems for which there is a general agreement about what needs to be done as opposed to adaptive problems where there is uncertainty and disagreement about what needs to be done.

In order to tackle adaptive problems Heifetz outlines a framework or set of processes that essentially involve the team or community where the problem is based and providing a safe yet challenging environment where people are encouraged to focus on creating a solution to the 'wicked' problem. There are clearly aspects of the approach that lend themselves to promoting innovation and as such may be useful to the challenges facing many health systems.

KEY ROLES OF MEDICAL LEADERS

Over the past decade there has been a steady growth in the number of designated medical leadership roles. We have discussed already how these roles have evolved, moving from a rather stuttering position where there was uncertainty about value of the roles and limited enthusiasm from those taking up these positions. Today effective performers in these roles are critical to system and organisational change.

Interestingly, despite the criticality of these roles, it is probable that most incumbents would have little direct relationship with the earlier debate about leadership models. Therefore, success (or otherwise) in the exercise of the roles has thus far been heavily dependent upon the personal qualities individuals bring to the position. It is vital for the future that a more professional approach to preparation is adopted involving systematic and sustained training for all clinicians in management and leadership. In this way the entire level of service delivery, change and innovation can be improved to meet the challenges ahead.

The introduction and implementation of the MLCF for all doctors will provide a basic platform of management and leadership skills but further specific training will be required as individuals move on to these formal positions. Currently there are a range of development provisions for such roles ranging from national and regional development programmes to individual university master's and MBA programmes. The National Leadership Council is currently seeking to create a structure that will enable individuals to move coherently from appropriate levels acquiring the specific and relevant skills en route. As the leadership task becomes more complex it will be essential that the technical expertise of the medical profession is brought together with the necessary management and leadership skills. As Mountford (2010) has suggested, never before has medical leadership been more essential and desirable.

REFERENCES

Alimo-Metcalfe B, Alban-Metcalfe T. The development of a new transformational leadership questionnaire. *Journal of Occupational and Organisational Psychology.* 2001; **74**: 1–27.

Darmer P. The subjectivity of management. *Journal of Organisational Change Management.* 2000; **13**(4): 1–15.

Grint K. Literature Review on Leadership. London: Cabinet Office; 2001.

Grint K. Management or leadership? *J Health Serv Res Policy.* 2002; **7**(4): 248–51.

Hartley J, Benington J. Leadership for Healthcare. Bristol: The Policy Press; 2010.

Heifetz R. *Leadership Without Easy Answers.* Cambridge, MA: Belknapp Press; 1994.

Higgs M. How can we make sense of leadership in the 21st century? *Leadership and Organisation Development Journal.* 2003; **24**(5): 1–17.

Houghton JD, Neck CP, Manz CC. Self-leadership and superleadership: the heart and art of creating shared leadership in Pearce. In: Pearce CL, Conger JA, editors. Shared Leadership: reframing the hows and whys of leadership. Thousand Oaks, CA: Sage Publications; 2002; 126–32.

Konu A, Viitanen E. Shared leadership in Finnish social and health care. *Leadership in Health Services.* 2008; **21**(1): 28–40.

Mountford J. Clinical leadership: bringing the strands together. In: Stanton E, Lemer C, Mountford J, editors. *Clinical Leadership: bridging the divide.* London: MA Healthcare; 2010.

Northouse PG. *Leadership: theory and practice.* London: Sage; 2010.

Pearce CL, Conger JA. *All Those Years Ago: the historical underpinnings of shared leadership.* In: Pearce CL, Conger JA, editors. *Shared Leadership: reframing the hows and whys of leadership.* Thousand Oaks, CA: Sage; 2003; 1–18.

Pearce CL, Manz CC, Sims Jr HP. Is shared leadership the key to team success? *Organisational Dynamics.* 2009; **38**(3): 234–8.

Spurgeon P, Cragg R. Is it management or leadership? In: Chambers R, Mohanna K, Spurgeon P, et al., editors. *How to Succeed as a Leader.* Oxford: Radcliffe Publishing; 2007.

Willcocks S. Doctors and leadership in the UK National Health Service. *Clinician in Management.* 2005; **13**: 11–21.

CHAPTER 4

Health system reform and the role of medical leaders

The aim of this chapter is to describe recent trends in healthcare reform in developed countries and the implications for medical leadership. The central argument advanced in the chapter is that there is a gap between the rhetoric and reality of reform in that the impact of many of the policies that have been pursued is more limited than promised or expected. The experience in England is used to illustrate this argument, drawing on the experience of the Griffiths Report, the internal market, the reforms implemented by New Labour and more recent initiatives from the Conservative-Liberal Democrat coalition government.

An explanation of the limited impact of healthcare reforms can be found in the nature of healthcare organisations as professional bureaucracies. With front-line staff – especially doctors – having considerable autonomy there is no certainty that policies promulgated at the top will be carried through in practice. A key feature of professional bureaucracies is the critical role played by leaders from professional backgrounds in making change happen. However, professional bureaucracies can be slow to change, indicating the important contribution of managers and policy-makers to performance improvement.

The lesson from healthcare reform is the need to combine top-down and bottom-up approaches. Change led from the top without the engagement of doctors and other clinical staff will tend to have a limited impact; equally, change led from the bottom will result in pockets of innovation rather than system-wide improvement. In the next stage of reform the challenge is to link professional leadership in healthcare organisations and clinical microsystems with system-wide leadership as part of a coherent strategy of improvement.

FOUR PHASES OF HEALTH REFORM

Governments have come to play a major role in the financing and provision of health services because of well-known market failures. These failures include information asymmetry between users and providers, risk selection by insurers, and moral hazard which has led to overuse of services by patients and oversupply of services by providers. Government intervention has resulted in public financing comprising the major portion of health service spending in most developed countries. It has also been associated with full or part public ownership of hospitals and healthcare facilities in many systems, and increasing public regulation of health insurers and providers.

Since at least the 1970s, there have been concerns about the effectiveness of government intervention in healthcare. This has given rise to a debate about government failure in healthcare as well as market failure and has resulted in an ongoing process of health reform as politicians seek to bring about improvements in health system performance. In a review of experience in a number of developed countries conducted in the mid 1990s, Ham (1997) described three main phases in this process, illustrated in Box 4.1.

Box 4.1 Trends in healthcare reform

PHASE ONE	Late 1970s/early 1980s
Theme	Cost containment at the macro level
Policy instruments	Prospective global budgets for hospitals Controls over hospital building and the acquisition of medical equipment Limits on doctor's fees and incomes Restrictions on the numbers undertaking education and training
PHASE TWO	Late 1980s/early 1990s
Theme	Micro efficiency and responsiveness to users
Policy instruments	Market-like mechanisms Management reforms Budgetary incentives
PHASE THREE	Late 1990s
Theme	Rationing and priority-setting
Policy instruments	Public health Primary care Managed care Health technology assessment Evidence-based medicine

Source: Reproduced from: Ham, editor. *Health Care Reform*. Maidenhead: Open University Press; 1997. Used with the kind permission of The Open University Press/McGraw-Hill Publishing Company.

The first phase focused on cost containment at the macro level and made use of various policy instruments, including prospective global budgets for hospitals, controls over hospital building and the acquisition of medical equipment, limits on doctors' fees and incomes, and restrictions on the numbers undertaking education and training for clinical roles.

The second phase was characterised by a concern to achieve increased efficiency and enhanced responsiveness at the micro level. It was at this point that there became growing interest in the use of market-like mechanisms within publicly funded systems, alongside reforms designed to strengthen the management of health services and introduce budgetary incentives to improve performance. The changes that followed from the Griffiths Report in the United Kingdom in 1983 and the subsequent internal market reforms promulgated by the Thatcher government exemplified the second phase of reform and were paralleled by similar developments in a number of other countries.

In the third phase of reform, attention shifted to healthcare rationing, or priority-setting. This reflected the financial constraints under which health systems operated during the 1990s and a concern to increase allocative efficiency and not just technical efficiency. Policy instruments adopted during this period included health technology assessment, the promotion of evidence-based medicine, and the use of expert committees to advise on priority setting. In parallel there was renewed interest in prevention and public health alongside attempts to strengthen the role of primary care. It was during this phase that managed care took hold in the United States, entailing restrictions on the choices of patients and doctors and increased scrutiny of clinical decisions.

In more recent times, a fourth phase of reform can be identified, focused on improving the quality and safety of healthcare. The concern with quality and safety arose out of increasing recognition of the 'quality chasm' in healthcare, described most comprehensively in a major study published by the United States Institute of Medicine (2001). Various policies characterised this phase, including initiatives to measure the outcomes of care and publish the results, the defining of desirable standards of care and the inspection of providers in relation to these standards, and the creation of new agencies with a specific focus on quality and safety. At the time of writing, the emphasis on quality and safety remains a work in progress, and is being pursued in parallel with reforms introduced in earlier phases.

In identifying these four phases of reform, two points should be emphasised. First, not all of these reforms were taken up in all countries; and national contexts and histories, as well as ideological factors and institutional arrangements, influenced the paths taken in different systems. Second, linked to this, while there were similarities in the policies adopted in some countries, there is little evidence to support the argument that healthcare systems were converging as a result of the reforms that were pursued (Marmor, Freeman, Okma, 2005). To be sure, there was increased interest in the initiatives developed in one system being taken up and adapted in others, but differences between system in forms of financing and delivery remained more important than similarities.

LESSONS LEARNED

Reviewing the experience of healthcare reform in different countries and variations in performance, the Organisation for Economic Co-operation and Development (OECD) has identified a number of lessons from international experience, noting that 'countries now know quite a bit about which tools and approaches can be used to accomplish many key policy objectives', while adding that these tools and approaches have been used 'with varying degrees of success' (OECD, 2004, p. 19). The OECD has also identified a number of promising directions for health policy in future, including:

- action to improve population health status and health outcomes, for example by investing more in prevention, tackling the determinants of ill health and developing quality indicators
- action to foster adequate and equitable access to care, for example by eliminating financial barriers to access
- action to increase health system responsiveness, for example by reducing waiting times for treatment and facilitating informed choice
- action to ensure sustainable costs and financing, for example through controls over payments, prices and the supply of services and the elimination of coverage for ancillary or luxury services
- action to increase the efficiency of health systems, for example by managing demand through gatekeepers and clinical prioritisation and technology assessment
- action to improve overall health system performance, for example through investment in health information technology and benchmarking performance against peers.

The work of the OECD, together with other reviews and assessments (Wallace, 2004); (Blank, Burau, 2007); (Gauld, 2009), underlines the complexity of health reform and the extent of unfinished business. It also demonstrates the uncertainties facing policymakers and the need to make trade-offs in pursuing different objectives.

One clear conclusion that can be drawn from experience since the 1970s is the gap between rhetoric and reality (Ham, 1997). While health reforms are often introduced with high expectations and with the promise of transformational results, their impact is usually more modest. If part of the explanation of the limited impact of reform is to be found in weaknesses in policy design, then equally important is the ability of front-line professionals to frustrate the intentions of reformers either through active resistance or simply failure to lend their support to new policies. Also important is the way in which the institutional logics of different systems mediate the reforming intentions of policymakers, as demonstrated by Tuohy in her comparative analysis of healthcare reform in Canada, the United Kingdom and the United States (Tuohy, 1999).

The response of governments in these circumstances is often to look for new directions of reform, resulting in hyperactivity in health policymaking. This is reinforced by frequent changes in the political parties controlling government with newly elected ministers wanting to show that they bring fresh thinking to their responsibilities. The experience of health reform in England offers a case in point.

HEALTH REFORM IN ENGLAND AS AN EXAMPLE

Health reform in England followed an incremental path until the election of the Thatcher government in 1979. The neoliberal instincts of the government, coupled with pressures on public spending, led to a series of efficiency initiatives being introduced in the NHS. At the heart of these initiatives was a concern to make the NHS more business-like by adopting the precepts of what became known as the new public management. This was exemplified by the Griffiths Report of 1983, commissioned by the government to advise on the management of the NHS and how it could be strengthened.

THE GRIFFITHS REPORT AND GENERAL MANAGEMENT

The report was produced by a small team, led by Roy Griffiths, deputy chairman and managing director of the Sainsbury's supermarket chain, and it offered a fundamental critique of NHS management and its failure to ensure that resources were used either efficiently or with the needs of patients in mind. Specifically, the report identified the absence of a clearly defined general management function as the main weakness of the NHS, commenting:

> 'Absence of this general management support means that there is no driving force seeking and accepting direct and personal responsibility for developing management plans, securing their implementation and monitoring actual achievement. It means that the process of devolution of responsibility, including discharging responsibility to the Units, is far too slow.' (Griffiths Report, 1983, p. 12)

Accordingly, the report recommended that general managers should be appointed at all levels in the NHS to provide leadership, introduce a continual search for change and cost improvement, motivate staff and develop a more dynamic management approach. At the same time, the report stated that hospital doctors 'must accept the management responsibility which goes with clinical freedom' (p. 18) and participate fully in decisions about priorities. Another key proposal was that the management of the NHS at the centre should be streamlined and strengthened through the establishment of a Health Services Supervisory Board and an NHS Management

Board, with the chairman of the management board being drawn from outside the NHS and the civil service. The team concluded:

> 'action is now badly needed and the Health Service can ill afford to indulge in any lengthy self-imposed Hamlet-like soliloquy as a precursor or alternative to the required action.' (p. 24)

This advice was heeded by the secretary of state who, in welcoming the report, announced that he accepted the general thrust of what the team had to say. Subsequently, the supervisory board and management board were established within the Department of Health and Social Security, and the government asked health authorities to appoint general managers at all levels in the service. The government also endorsed the Griffiths Report's view that doctors should be involved in management and that they should be given responsibility for management budgets. To this end, a number of demonstration projects were established, and in 1986 management budgeting was superseded by the resource management initiative. The change in terminology signalled a shift in emphasis away from the development of a budgeting system in isolation towards an approach in which doctors and nurses took on more responsibility for the management of resources as a whole.

Research evidence indicates that the impact of these changes was mixed. As far as the changes in the Department of Health and Social Security were concerned, Griffiths' own assessment was that they were 'half hearted in their implementation' (Griffiths, 1992, p. 65) and did not succeed in introducing the clarity he and his team had sought. At a local level, the impact of general management varied, with some studies arguing that managers had gained influence in relation to doctors and others maintaining that change had been minimal (Harrison, 1994). In relation to resource management, an evaluation indicated that some progress had been made in involving doctors and nurses in management, but much remained to be done and the process of change could not be rushed (Packwood, Keen, Buxton, 1991). The most important effect of the Griffiths Report was to lay the foundations for the introduction of the internal market in 1991 through the appointment of a cadre of chief executives within the NHS who were largely receptive to the policies that were being pursued. We explore the impact of Griffiths Report and the Resource Management Initiative on medical leadership in more detail in Chapter 5.

THE INTERNAL MARKET

The Thatcher government's plans to introduce an internal market within the NHS were a direct response to the funding crisis that emerged in the late 1980s. With NHS organisations finding it difficult to balance their budgets in the face of increasing demands for their services, the government allocated additional funding to the NHS and at the same time established a far-reaching review of the future of the NHS led by the Prime Minister. As the review progressed, it became clear that there was little enthusiasm for a major change in how the NHS was financed. The reasons for this included support for taxation as the principal method of funding and recognition that the alternatives all had drawbacks and might not help in addressing the problems that gave rise to the review.

With the financing debate taking a back seat, greater attention was paid to how resources could be used more efficiently through changes to the delivery of health services. Of particular importance was the proposal that hospitals should compete for resources in an internal market. This proposal had originally been advocated by Alain Enthoven in 1985 (Enthoven, 1985), and it was taken up and developed by right-wing think tanks such as the Adam Smith Institute and the Centre for Policy Studies. The debate about delivery also included proposals to make doctors more accountable for their performance and to involve doctors more effectively in management. In parallel, suggestions were put forward for strengthening the management of health services by building on the introduction of general management.

The plans to create an internal market were set out in detail in the white paper, Working for Patients (Secretary of State for Health *et al.*, 1989). These plans entailed separating the functions of health authorities in order to create a clear distinction between purchasers and providers. As purchasers of care for their populations, health authorities were expected to negotiate contracts with services provided by self-governing NHS Trusts and directly managed units. In parallel, general practitioners were offered the opportunity to take on a budget to buy care for their patients under the general practitioner fundholding scheme. The principal aim of separating purchaser and provider roles was to create the conditions for hospitals and other providers to compete for patients, thereby providing the stimulus to improve performance that the government felt was lacking.

Researchers have offered a variety of judgements on the impact of the internal market. The most thorough analysis of the evidence concluded that overall little change – positive or negative – could be detected (Le Grand, Mays, Mulligan, 1998). This analysis systematically reviewed the findings from a large number of research studies, seeking to assess the impact of the reforms under five broad headings: efficiency, equity, quality, choice and responsiveness and accountability. Like other researchers, these authors emphasised the difficulty of separating the effects of the reforms from other changes in policy occurring at the same time and from increases in NHS funding. Given this caveat, they noted some evidence of improvements in efficiency, indications that equity was affected adversely by the differential access achieved by GP fundholders, no evidence that trust status had an impact on quality, minimal change to choice and responsiveness, and no real difference in accountability arrangements.

Le Grand and colleagues emphasised that their analysis was concerned primarily with *measurable* change, and they added that there was some evidence of cultural change as a result of the reforms, which may not have been adequately captured in the research studies they reviewed. In relation to cultural change, the findings of

Ferlie and colleagues lend support to the argument that *Working for Patients* did have an impact on roles and relationships within the NHS (Ferlie *et al.*, 1996). Among the changes reported by these researchers was a reorientation of hospital specialists towards GPs and some evidence that the influence of managers and of clinicians in management roles was increasing. These findings echo the author's own assessment based both on research into the reforms and experience of working with a wide range of NHS bodies throughout this period (Ham, 1996, 1997). Yet even allowing for these effects, the impact of the internal market fell short of the expectations that had accompanied its introduction.

NEW LABOUR AND THE NHS

Health reform in England took a further turn following the election of a Labour government under Tony Blair in 1997. Voted into office on a platform that included a commitment to abolish the internal market, New Labour as it became known focused initially on using targets and performance management to implement its objectives in areas of high priority such as access to care. This included developing national service frameworks in areas of high clinical priority, for example heart disease and cancer, and setting up the National Institute for Clinical Excellence to offer guidance on the use of drugs and other technologies. A major aim in adopting these approaches was to reduce the so-called 'postcode lottery' within the NHS by ensuring much greater consistency of service provision across the country. Additional funding was allocated to the NHS to support implementation of the government's plans, and much of this funding was used to buy extra capacity in order to reduce waiting lists and waiting times for treatment.

Subsequently, the government devolved responsibility for budgets to primary care trusts at a local level and enabled high-performing NHS trusts to become NHS Foundation Trusts no longer in a line management relationship with the Secretary of State for Health. These policies formed the basis of a reintroduction of market-like mechanisms from 2002 onwards in response to recognition that there were limits to how far government could achieve improvements in performance through targets and performance management. New Labour's plans for competition and choice were in many ways more radical than those of the Thatcher government, involving a bigger role for the independent sector, greater autonomy for NHS providers, and a funding system in which money really did follow patients. Steps were taken too to promote higher standards of care by strengthening the regulation of the NHS and the independent sector through the establishment of the Commission for Health Improvement and its successors. Improving the quality of care and patient safety was also the core theme of the final report of the NHS Next Stage review led by Lord Darzi (Secretary of State for Health, 2008).

Various organisations have evaluated the impact of New Labour's reforms. The Nuffield Trust's assessment of the impact of the reforms on healthcare quality (Leatherman, Sutherland, 2008) noted major improvements in the quality of care but argued that these improvements had not been commensurate with the investment that had occurred. A number of explanations were offered for this, including an ideological rift between advocates of central control and supporters of devolution within the NHS; a predisposition to structural change and reorganisation with adverse consequences for staff morale; a tendency to promote new policies as 'flavour of the month'; perennial problems with coordination of care, duplication of effort and territorialism; strong policy conceptualisation that was unmatched by the requisite competence in implementation; and deficiencies in availability of data to report on quality improvement.

The assessment prepared by the Audit Commission and the Healthcare Commission (2008) focused particularly on progress with the implementation of the government's market-oriented reforms. This assessment gave the government credit for significant progress in improving the performance of the NHS, as evidenced by much shorter waiting times and other improvements summarised in the Healthcare Commission's annual health check. However, it noted that progress had resulted mainly from increases in funding and the use of national targets, rather than the market-oriented reforms introduced by the Blair government. There was no evidence that patient choice had had a significant impact, the results achieved by NHS Foundation Trusts were not striking, and commissioning remained a weak link in the reform programme.

Although noting that some of the reforms had been implemented too recently to enable a proper assessment to be made, and that the programme as a whole had potential for the future, the Audit Commission and the Healthcare Commission concluded that there were a number of barriers to further progress, including the need to engage staff more effectively in the process of change. This recommendation was echoed in the final report of the NHS Next Stage Review led by Lord Darzi, which argued strongly for reform to be led locally with the full engagement of clinicians and other front-line staff. The Conservative-Liberal Democrat coalition government elected in 2010 has gone further in arguing that the empowerment of clinical staff should be a cornerstone of the NHS in future, especially through GPs and primary care teams taking control of budgets. The coalition government is also cutting management costs and abolishing strategic health authorities and primary care trusts in the belief that this will remove bureaucratic controls and free up front-line staff to lead improvements in care.

THE IMPLEMENTATION GAP AND MEDICAL LEADERSHIP

The story of health reform in England in the last three decades is a story of a permanent revolution in which governments have used a wide variety of policies in the hope of improving performance. It is also a story of big bang changes that have delivered less than they have promised. The gap between policy intention and impact is not unique to England and similar accounts could be written about the experience of other countries.

In relation to the Griffiths Report and general management, the internal market, and New Labour's reforms, there is explicit recognition of the need to involve doctors more effectively in management and leadership roles, even though this was not the main aim of reform in any of these periods. Only in Lord Darzi's final report is clinical leadership identified as central to health reform, and it is probably no accident that it required a report written by a health minister from a medical background to acknowledge the importance of clinical leadership. The point to emphasise here is that policymakers can prod and poke healthcare systems as much as they like, but their ability to make change happen is mediated by the autonomy afforded to healthcare professionals delivering care to patients at the front line. The same point has been put rather differently by Klein (2006), who has noted that the exclusion of doctors from a major role in policymaking has not weakened their ability to shape the implementation of policy and because of that they retain considerable influence over the direction of the NHS.

An explanation of this can be found in the work of organisational theorists such as Henry Mintzberg, who characterises healthcare organisations as professional bureaucracies rather than machine bureaucracies (Mintzberg, 1979). One of the characteristics of professional bureaucracies is that front-line staff members have a large measure of control over the content of work by virtue of their training and specialist knowledge. Consequently, hierarchical directives issued by those nominally in control often have limited impact, and indeed may be resisted by front-line staff. In this respect, as in others, professional bureaucracies are different from machine bureaucracies (such as government departments).

More specifically, they have an inverted power structure in which staff members at the bottom of the organisation generally have greater influence over decision-making on a day-to-day basis than staff in formal positions of authority. It follows that organisational leaders have to negotiate rather than impose new policies and practices, working in a way that is sensitive to the culture of these organisations. The following observation from a study of the impact of business process reengineering in an English hospital summarises the challenge in this way:

> 'Significant change in clinical domains cannot be achieved without the co-operation and support of clinicians. . . . . Clinical support is associated with process redesign that resonates with clinical agendas related to patient care, services development and professional development. . . . To a large degree interesting doctors in re-engineering involves persuasion that is often informal, one consultant at a time, and interactive over time . . . clinical commitment to change, ownership of change and support for change constantly need to be checked, reinforced and worked on'
> (Bowns, McNulty, 1999, 66–7)

As this observation suggests, control in professional bureaucracies is achieved primarily through horizontal rather than vertical processes. These processes are driven by professionals themselves who use collegial influences to secure co-ordination of work. In healthcare organisations, professional networks play an important role in ensuring control and co-ordination, both within and between organisations, alongside peer review and peer pressure. Collegial influences depend critically on the credibility of the professionals at their core, rather than the power of people in formal positions of authority.

Three implications for leadership follow. First, in professional bureaucracies, professionals play key leadership roles, both informally and where they are appointed to formal positions. Much more so than in machine bureaucracies, the background of leaders and their standing among peers have a major bearing on their ability to exercise effective leadership, and to bring about change.

Second, professional bureaucracies are characterised by dispersed or distributed leadership. In healthcare organisations, clinical microsystems (Batalden *et al.*, 2003) are a particularly important focus for leadership. It follows that in professional bureaucracies there is a need for large numbers of leaders from clinical backgrounds at different levels. A focus on leadership only at the top or most senior levels risks missing a central feature of these bureaucracies.

Third, much of the evidence highlights the importance of collective leadership in healthcare organisation. Collective leadership has two dimensions: first, it refers to the role of leadership teams rather than charismatic individuals; and second, it draws attention to the need to bring together constellations of leaders at different levels when major change programmes are undertaken, as demonstrated by empirical research into leadership in Canadian hospitals undertaken by Jean-Louis Denis and his colleagues (Denis *et al.*, 2001).

To draw out these implications is to underscore not just the nature of leadership in professional bureaucracies but also the importance of 'followership'. Put simply, the large measure of control that front-line staff members have over the content of work can result in professional bureaucracies becoming disconnected hierarchies or even organised anarchies. Appointing respected and experienced professionals to leadership roles is often advocated as the response to this challenge. Chantler is one of the foremost advocates of this approach, arguing that in Guy's Hospital:

> '*By giving significant responsibility for the organisation to those who actually delivered the service, we aimed to reduce the disconnection that occurs in hospitals, as pointed out by Mintzberg, between those at the top who organise the strategy and those at the service end who deliver care to patients*' (Chantler, 1999, p. 1179)

However, in itself this may not be sufficient to address the need for control, co-ordination and innovation. As well, healthcare organisations have increasingly recognised the requirement to strengthen the role of all staff as followers; Silversin and Kornacki (2000) emphasise this in their work on medical leadership in the United States and argue that organisations should invest in organisation development and not just leadership development.

NECESSARY BUT NOT SUFFICIENT

The other point to emphasise is that hospitals and primary care organisations comprise conservatives as well as innovators and in Mintzberg's terms are often slow to change. This means that left to their own devices, these organisations may not adapt quickly enough to meet rising public expectations. As a consequence, at the same time as greater efforts need to be made to involve professionals in leadership roles, the contribution of managers and policymakers to health system performance improvement has to be recognised. This does not mean advocacy of further big bang reforms whose impact has often been limited. Rather, it calls for a more nuanced approach in which managers work with professionals to make change happen, and policymakers pay more attention than hitherto in engaging professionals themselves in bringing about improvement, as Lord Darzi has proposed.

Examples discussed in detail elsewhere in this book (*see* Chapter 6) such as Kaiser Permanente and Mayo Clinic illustrate in practical terms how high-performing organisations have developed effective partnerships between doctors and managers. In England, the implementation of service line reporting (in many ways the successor to management budgeting and resource management) in NHS Foundation Trusts is based on similar principles and early evidence indicates promising results from this approach. Under service line reporting, hospital services are organised into distinct and relevant business units, and each unit is able to compare the cost of providing services with the income it earns. Service line reporting depends critically on leadership by doctors and managers, the provision of timely information about the performance of services, and incentives to motivate staff to improve performance. In one example, this resulted in a general surgery service line in an NHS Foundation Trust in the northeast of England converting a deficit of £1 million into a small surplus (Ham, 2009a).

While there are fewer examples of policymakers engaging professionals in bringing about improvement, experience in England with the appointment of national clinical directors or tsars is again relevant. National clinical directors are senior and experienced doctors appointed by the government to lead the development of services in major areas of clinical priority like cancer and cardiac care. The progress made in improving the performance of these services has resulted from the promulgation of national service frameworks, the allocation of additional funding, the use of targets to specify the priorities to be pursued and the leadership provided by the national clinical directors. To make this point is of course to emphasise that performance improvement in healthcare is the result of many factors and to caution against explanations that focus on one of these factors at the expense of others. As Ferlie and Shortell (2001) have argued in their analysis of quality improvement in healthcare, action is needed at different levels – individual, microsystem, organisational and larger system – and on a range of variables if improvement is to move beyond pockets of innovation and have a wider impact.

The important conclusion this leads to is that medical leadership within clinical microsystems and healthcare organisations may be a necessary condition of health service improvement, but it is not sufficient. The challenge in the next stage of healthcare reform is to combine top-down and bottom-up approaches in recognition that one without the other is likely to have limited effects. This conclusion is underlined by experience from other sectors, suggesting that successful change requires action on several fronts simultaneously as well as the need to work across a series of dualities (Pettigrew, 1999). These dualities include not only linking top-down and bottom-up but also promoting the standardisation of care where there is evidence this will bring benefits and ensuring that services are customised around the needs of individuals; using competition in some areas of service provision and promoting cooperation in others; and working through the hierarchy to achieve change while also facilitating the emergence of networks.

Working across these dualities and leading change across several fronts simultaneously calls for political skills of a much high order than have often been apparent in healthcare systems in the past. This is a big 'ask' given that politicians in stewardship roles in healthcare are often inexperienced in leading large-scale change and impatient to see results (Ham, 2009b). As Ham argued in a paper published in the Lancet:

> '. . . the role of reformers is less to search for the next eye-catching idea than to build the capacity for change and innovation to occur from within health care organisations. Building the capacity of people and organisations to bring about improvements might be slow and unglamorous work, but in the longer term it is likely to have a bigger effect than further bold policy strokes. Policy makers and managers also have a role on provision of systems and institutional leadership and framing of the agenda for reform. The trick that has to be accomplished is to harness the energies of clinicians and reformers in the quest for improvements in performance that benefit patients. Succeeding with this trick needs reformers to develop a better appreciation of the organisations they are striving to change, and clinicians to acknowledge that change is needed. The importance of linking top down and bottom up approaches to improvement has never been greater. On this link, nothing less than the future of organised health care systems depends' (Ham, 2003).

CONCLUSION

Experience of healthcare reform since the 1970s highlights the need to engage doctors more effectively in the process of reform at all levels. This includes making greater efforts to develop medical leadership in microsystems, healthcare organisations, and at the systems level. The ability of front-line staff in professional bureaucracies to frustrate the intentions of reformers means that the leadership provided by policymakers and managers needs to be joined with the commitment of doctors and other clinicians to improve the quality of care for patients on a system-wide basis. One without the other is bound to lead to further partial implementation of healthcare reforms and increasing frustration on the part of both reformers and those who feel reform is being done to them.

REFERENCES

Audit Commission and The Healthcare Commission. *Is the Treatment Working? Progress with the NHS System Reform Programme.* London: Audit Commission; 2008.

Batalden PB, Nelson E, Mohr J, *et al.* (2003) Microsystems in Health Care: Part 5. How Leaders are Leading. *Jt Comm J Qual Saf.* 2003; **29**(6): 297–308.

Blank RH, Burau V. *Comparative Health Policy.* Houndmills: Palgrave Macmillan; 2004.

Bowns I, McNulty T. *Reengineering Leicester Royal Infirmary: an independent evaluation of implementation and impact.* Sheffield: School of Health and Related Research, University of Sheffield; 1999.

Chantler C. The role and education of doctors in the delivery of health care. *Lancet.* 1999; **353**(9159): 1178–81.

Denis J, Lamothe L, Langley A. The dynamics of collective leadership and strategic change in pluralistic organisations. *Academy of Management Journal.* 2001; **44**: 809–937.

Department of Health. *The NHS Next Stage Review: high quality care for all.* London: HMSO; 2008.

Enthoven A. *Reflections on the Management of the NHS.* London: Nuffield Provincial Hospitals Trust; 1985.

Ferlie E, Ashburner L, Fitzgerald L, *et al. The New Public Management in Action.* Oxford: Oxford University Press; 1996.

Ferlie E, Shortell S. Improving the quality of health care in the United Kingdom and the United States: a framework for change. *The Millbank Quarterly.* 2001; **70**: 281–315.

Gauld R. *The New Health Policy.* Maidenhead: Open University Press; 2009.

Griffiths R. Seven years of progress – general management in the NHS. *Health Economics.* 1992; **1**(1): 61–70.

Griffiths Report. *NHS Management Inquiry.* London: HMSO; 1983.

Ham C. *Public, Private or Community: what next for the NHS?* London: Demos; 1996.

Ham C, editor. *Health Care Reform.* Buckingham: Open University Press; 1997.

Ham C. *Management and Competition in the NHS.* Abingdon: Radcliffe Medical Press; 1997.

Ham C. Improving the performance of health services: the role of clinical leadership. *Lancet.* 2003; **361**(9373): 1978–80.

Ham C. *Health in a Cold Climate: developing an intelligent response to the financial challenges facing the NHS.* London: The Nuffield Trust; 2009a.

Ham C. *Health Policy in Britain.* 6th ed. Basingstoke: Macmillan; 2009b.

Harrison S. *National Health Service Management in the 1980s.* Aldershot: Avebury; 1994.

Institute of Medicine. *Crossing the Quality Chasm: a new health system for the 21st century.* Washington: National Academy Press; 2001.

Klein R. *The New Politics of the NHS.* 5th ed. New York, NY: Longman; 2006.

Le Grand J, Mays N, Mulligan J, editors. *Learning from the NHS Internal Market*. London: The King's Fund; 1998.

Leatherman S, Sutherland K. *The Quest for Quality: refining the NHS reforms*. London: The Nuffield Trust; 2008.

Marmor T, Freeman R, Okma K. Comparative perspectives and policy learning in the world of health care. *Journal of Comparative Policy Analysis*. 2005; **7**(4): 331–48.

Mintzberg H. *The Structuring of Organisations*. Englewood Cliffs: Prentice-Hall; 1979.

OECD. *Towards High-Performing Health Systems*. Paris: OECD; 2004.

Packwood T, Keen J, Buxton M. *Hospitals in Transition*. Milton Keynes: Open University Press; 1991.

Pettigrew A. Organising to improve company performance. *Warwick Business School Hot Topics*. 1999; **1**(5). Available at: www.wbs.ac.uk/downloads/hot_topics/hot_topics_06.pdf (accessed 21 April 2011).

Secretary of State for Health *et al*. *Working for Patients*. London: HMSO; 1989.

Silversin J, Kornacki M. *Leading Physicians Through Change*. Tampa: American College of Physician Executives; 2000.

Tuohy C. *Accidental Logics: the dynamics of change in the health care arena in the United States, Britain and Canada*. New York, NY: Oxford University Press; 1999.

Wallace P. The health of nations. *Economist*. 17 July 2004.

CHAPTER 5

A historical perspective on medical leadership

As Chapter 4 has demonstrated, experience of healthcare reform since the 1970s has stressed the need to engage doctors more effectively in the process of reform. This need has been strongly reinforced by the current emphasis on health reform being led locally by clinicians.

This chapter outlines the way in which doctors have been involved in management, leadership and transformation of services over the past 60 years since the inception of the NHS in 1948. It can perhaps best be summarised as a movement from major domination preceding the NHS through a period of disenfranchisement immediately thereafter, right through until closer to the 1974 reorganisation of the NHS. By this time a few doctors, generally reluctantly, accepted representative roles. However, the latter decades of the 20th century and the early years of this century have led to doctors playing an increasing role in management, leadership and transformation of services at all levels of the NHS.

It is always tempting to analyse or assess one particular health policy announcement or intervention as a radical change from the status quo. Far more often, it is a small partial adjustment or incremental change from the current position. Nevertheless, if reviewed from a longer-term perspective, it is likely to be an important step in a more fundamental strategic journey that, over time, leads to significant change in paradigms or philosophies.

The current focus on medical leadership as particularly espoused by *High Quality Care for All: Next Stage Review (2008)* is perhaps a further step in the journey of the changing role of doctor in the NHS since its inception in 1948. This has been reinforced by the Conservative-Liberal Democrat coalition government's intention to give health professionals greater decision-making powers. As this book was going to press, the government published its White Paper '*Equity and excellence: liberating the NHS*' (2010). The new policy direction outlined in the White Paper reinforces the important role of medical leaders across the health system but particularly within the proposed GP consortia.

MEDICAL DISENFRANCHISEMENT: THE EARLY YEARS OF THE NHS

As the NHS and many other systems internationally seek to get more doctors involved in management, it is worth reflecting that the creation of the NHS in 1948 had created a framework within which medical professionals could become salaried employees whilst retaining clinical freedom.

Paton *et al.* contend:

'The compromise that brought medical consultants into the NHS resulted in the application of the existing consultants' contract, and the arrangement whereby medical consultants contracts were held in the 'remote filing cabinets' of Regional Hospital Boards (subsequently Regional Health Authorities). This was a clear signal to the medical profession that they were different from any other employee within the NHS, whose contract of employment was held at more local level' (Paton et al., 2005, p. 28).

This view is confirmed by Klein, who comments that:

'Implicit in the structure of the NHS was a bargain between the State and the medical profession. While central government controlled the budget, doctors controlled what happened within that budget. Financial power was concentrated at the centre; clinical power was concentrated at the periphery. Politicians in Cabinet made the decisions about how much to spend; doctors made the decision about which patient should get what kind of treatment' (Klein, 2006, p. 61).

As the independence of clinicians has eroded over the past few decades and with increasing regulation and accountability for performance it is interesting to note that only 20 years ago Strong and Robinson argued that, as a result of this deal, the NHS was 'fundamentally syndicalist in nature' (1990, p. 15) in that the medical profession was able to control and regulate its own activities without interference from politicians or managers.

Whilst the power-base of the medical profession is changing rapidly, the historical medicalisation of the process of healthcare has given doctors considerable power both in the doctor-patient relationship and in the relative subservience of the other healthcare professions. This imbalance has had a significant impact on the way doctors relate to their organisation and involvement in management of services.

This book provides evidence of the rapidly changing culture of NHS organisations and how the medical profession is changing. However, a number of quotes capture a sense of the medical culture during the latter years of the 20th century, e.g.:

'The moment you become a consultant (in Britain), you are omnipotent. You don't have to pay attention to your colleagues; you don't have to pay attention to anybody.'
                    Emeritus Professor of Surgery (in: Rosenthal, 1995)

'Doctors must play a bigger part in managing the health service to protect their clinical freedom.'

Professor Cyril Chantler (BMJ, 1989)

'Doctors are potentially the best managers in the health service. They have the longest and the best education of all those in the hospitals, the most experience, and are responsible for most of the decisions that lead to expenditure.'

Sir Anthony Grabham (BMJ, 1989)

As Pollard (2001) comments, these are somewhat protective and defensive views, as if noting a threat on the horizon (as subsequently realised) but one which could be safely navigated.

As Spurgeon (2001) summarised:

'The historical precedents that created the medical power base led initially to doctors existing in a closed sub-culture cushioned from scrutiny and challenge from others within the system. The individualistic culture affirmed by doctors' training served to support and reinforce this position. The public, too, were keen to endorse such an individual focus, believing that doctors should be concerned primarily with their patients and that health care organisations had some sort of secondary existence for the purpose of facilitating medical activity.'

Following the start of the NHS in July 1948, many hospitals were led by a medical superintendent supported by a matron and hospital administrator. A large number of general practitioners worked single-handedly. The responsibility for organising clinical services tended to reside with a plethora of local and regional medical advisory committees.

It is interesting to note that, as many hospitals now are questioning the role of medical staff committees, back in 1953 the Ministry of Health issued a circular (1953) outlining the Minister's view on the functions and constitution of Medical Staff Committees.

This was an important stage in the medical engagement journey for the NHS as it provided a clear message as to the importance of engaging doctors in advising and contributing to the running of both hospitals and groups of hospitals.

As Merivale states:

'The detailed arrangements for these committees in the majority of hospital groups are probably more rooted in past local history and customs than in the advice given in this circular with the result that arrangements are found to vary widely from group to group. Their effectiveness and the good relations or otherwise which they induce between the authority and its medical and dental staff vary equally widely. Indeed it could be argued in this matter that success may depend as much on tradition, personalities or even chance as upon organisation' (Merivale, 1969, p. 172–3).

Nevertheless, medical advisory and staff committees did become important forums for discussing medical matters. Lay hospital administrators quickly understood the risk of attempting to make decisions on such matters without due deference to the appropriate medical committee. Whilst the hospital administrator was generally invited (often to take minutes!), it was also not unusual for the administrator to be asked to leave the meeting whilst matters of medical sensitivity were discussed by the doctors only.

It is not the intention of this chapter to offer a detailed history lesson of the various organisational changes and their impact on managerial arrangements between 1948 and 1974. However, in terms of what was to follow from 1974 it was, in retrospect, a relatively dormant era in the policy history of the NHS.

Nevertheless, the role of doctors in contributing to the running of hospitals became an increasing issue during the 1960s and early 1970s and indeed became a significant theme of the 1974 reorganisation.

MEDICAL REPRESENTATION: THE COGWHEEL YEARS

A Joint Working Party on the Organisation of Medical Work in Hospitals was set up in 1965 to review the progress of the NHS particularly hospital services. The Working Party produced three reports between 1967 and 1974. Based on the design of the cover, they became known as the Cogwheel Reports.

These reports have had a significant impact on the way in which hospital services are organised internally over the past 40 years. Essentially, a system involving divisions of specialities was established, with representatives of the medical staff from the various specialties with responsibility to appraise their services and methods of provision.

Most hospitals established (as a minimum) divisions of: surgery, medicine, pathology, obstetrics and gynaecology, paediatrics, radiology and anaesthetics.

The chair of each of the divisions was generally elected by his or her peers for a period of two to four years. There was a tendency for the role to be given on seniority and often reluctantly undertaken on the basis of 'my turn'. There was no additional remuneration for the role and certainly no assessment of leadership capability.

As Levitt *et al.* report:

> 'Most hospital groups gradually implemented this scheme and by 1972 the second report was able to identify the essential elements of an effective Cogwheel system and to report that in large acute hospitals particularly, the system had been helpful in dealing with improved communications, reductions of in-patient waiting lists and the progressive control of medical expenditure' (Levitt et al., 1999, p. 172).

Put another way, Cogwheel divisions were there to cope with the problems of management that arose in the clinical field.

As we shall see later on, the Cogwheel system provided the platform for the subsequent phases of organisational arrangements within hospitals and the ways in which doctors are engaged in decision-making. However, the Cogwheel system still reinforced the position that the actions of doctors could not be directly controlled by managers.

It also should be noted that, with the exception of teaching hospitals, consultants were not employed by individual hospitals or by groups of hospitals but by the regional hospital boards. This did not change until around 1990.

The Cogwheel medical structure was the embryo of the clinical directorate system that followed, but as Paton *et al.* (2005) argue, with one fundamental difference – they had no resources to manage. At this stage in the life of the NHS it was not possible to apportion the global allocation into individual specialty budgets.

MEDICAL REPRESENTATION: THE GRIFFITHS DIRECTORATE WAY

Whilst many NHS Trusts are now embarking on internal strategies that see directorates as business units, the development of specialty budgets began as part of a demonstration project on management budgeting and was strongly reinforced by Sir Roy Griffiths in his inquiry into the management of the NHS, which was published in October 1983 (Griffiths Report, 1983). It was further endorsed by the Resource Management Initiative in 1986.

As we argue in Chapter 4, the Griffiths Inquiry is perhaps the tipping point in the modern history of doctors' greater involvement in the management and leadership of the NHS at all levels. It led to the introduction of general management throughout the NHS and perhaps more significantly the start of the transition from medical representation (Cogwheel system) to one slowly but surely based on medical leadership through the emerging clinical directorate system.

As Chantler (1994) stressed,

> 'This involvement by clinicians in management has to embrace a contribution both to the strategic and operational management of the service, in hospital, in the community, in practice, and in the commissioning role at district and central level, rather than doctors simply seeing themselves as there to give advice. That if you like, was the old role of the Medical Advisory Committee, functioning as a sort of Greek chorus, commenting on what was going on on the stage, but not taking part in the play' (Chantler, 1994, p. 17).

Just as Lord Darzi stressed the importance of clinical leadership in his clinical visions for the NHS in *High Quality Care for All* (2008), so Sir Roy Griffiths some 25 years earlier had recognised that to effect real improvement in productivity and quality required greater involvement of doctors. Put simply, the latter could not see how a service, department or organisation could be managed effectively unless it was managed by those who commit the resources.

It is also worth noting that this greater involvement of clinicians in the mid-1980s coincided with the drive for improved financial and activity information. It also came at a time when the NHS started to have a much higher political and media profile with many of its apparent failings being vigorously highlighted to the public on a regular basis.

Paton *et al.* (2005) suggest that the availability of relatively good information was a major stimulus in the evolution of doctors into management. They believe this was because it gave doctors the incentive of having resources to manage and use at local level. As Griffiths argued, hospital doctors 'must accept the management responsibility which goes with clinical freedom' (Griffiths Report, 1983, p. 18).

Most NHS hospitals began to introduce a medical management system based around clinical directorates. These tended initially to be similar specialty groupings to the previous Cogwheel divisions. Senior doctors were appointed as clinical directors responsible for leading the work of different services and specialties within the hospital. Many of the previous chairs of the Cogwheel divisions succeeded into clinical director roles. Little attention was given to the competences required of such role-holders, with more attention being given to tenure and structural arrangement. The vast majority had no prior training for the role and indeed for many years thereafter this continued, apart from some programmes offered by the British Association of Medical Managers (BAMM); a number of universities, e.g. Birmingham, Keele and Manchester; The King's Fund and other providers. A small number of enlightened hospitals initiated in-house programmes. Overall, whatever development provided to medical leaders tended to be ad hoc, variable and remedial.

Clinical directors combined their management and leadership roles with their clinical duties. Unlike the Cogwheel chair positions, clinical directors were often paid an additional session or two; most preferring to accept this increase in pay rather than reduce their clinical commitments. Furthermore, with financial constraints impeding the appointment of new consultants during the 1990s, chief executives were happy to accept no reduction in clinical sessions as well as gaining a clinical director with responsibilities for resource management.

Clinical directors usually worked with a nurse manager and business manager in a directorate team known as a tripartite team or triumvirate. Clinical directors were often part of the hospital executive team, creating a much stronger medical voice in both operational and strategic decision-making.

In addition to the appointment of clinical directors, hospitals appointed a medical director. The vast majority of these were again appointed on the basis of seniority, willingness, interest, etc., and not on any formal assessment of leadership competence or indeed by competition. Initially, most medical directors did not accept any reduction in clinical sessions and were offered additional sessions in recognition of their leadership activities.

The clinician prepared to accept a leadership role was therefore someone who, in effect, sat between two systems. One of these systems included the collegial and clinical professional environment where the doctor was an advocate for his/her colleagues whilst on the other hand being required to take a wider view of the clinical specialty and organisation. In the latter role the clinical director was involved in shaping the future direction using his or her clinical knowledge and experience with managers who were accountable, ultimately to politicians (Simpson, 2002). As Hopkinson argued, this wearing many hats is extremely difficult, forcing a clinician, '. . . at one moment to represent a clinical discipline and then ten minutes later to disadvantage that discipline to the greater corporate need of another area of the Trust or NHS at large' (Hopkinson, 2000, p. 5).

Guy's Hospital in London perhaps led the way in pioneering a new approach to medical leadership during the late 1980s and early 1990s based on the experience of the Johns Hopkins Hospital in the United States.

As Chantler (1990) acknowledged, there had to be an acceptance by the clinicians of the reality of cash limits, stressing that within them all have the ethical responsibility to ensure that resources are spent wisely to ensure effectiveness and efficiency. In a contribution to a report prepared by the Royal College of Physicians he also espoused a new philosophy that:

> 'where money is limited, profligacy in the care of one patient may lead to the denial of care of another. There must be constant attention to improving efficiency in economic terms and ensuring the effectiveness of treatment to produce the best outcome' (Royal College of Physicians, 1993, p. 3).

The Clinical Directorate model became the established internal management arrangement for hospitals in the NHS throughout the late 1980s and 1990s, particularly as the new policy strategy of the internal market became established during the latter period.

The Griffiths Report and its impact in starting a long-term process of renegotiating the role of clinicians in management and leadership and contributing to the emergence of a new definition of the medical profession cannot be underestimated. While some hospitals made progress in using clinical directorates to engage doctors in leadership roles and to achieve improvements in performance, others experienced difficulties. These difficulties are starkly illustrated in a detailed study of leadership in an NHS hospital in the 1990s undertaken by Bate (2000).

In this hospital, consultants did not accept the legitimacy of management, and as a result were able to undermine managerial power. The hospital was characterised by subcultures centred on microsystems that were isolated from each other. This was problematic when change was attempted involving more than one microsystem, as it led to tensions and often gridlock. Doctors held power and managers became afraid to challenge doctors lest they should face a vote of no confidence. Progress only became possible when doctors and managers agreed to establish a 'network community' (p. 504) in place of the system of clinical directorates which was seen to have been 'a failed experiment' (p. 509).

A more mixed picture emerged from a survey of clinical directorates in Scotland conducted by McKee and colleagues. This survey found wide variations in the way directorates were constructed and conducted their business. Three major directorates were identified (McKee, Marnoch, Dinnie, 1999). The dominant type, described as 'traditionalist', was characterised by a strong focus on operational issues and limited scope for innovation and change. Relationships between clinical directors and clinical colleagues remained embedded in a collegiate clinical network and were based on consensus building and facilitation.

The second type was described as 'managerialist' and was characterised by a business-oriented approach more in line with the philosophy of the Griffiths Report. Clinical directors in managerialist directorates had direct links with top managers in the hospital and were better placed to influence overall strategy and direction than those in traditionalist directorates. The third type was described as 'power-sharing' and involved clinical directors working across established specialty boundaries and operating as a team with the business manager and nurse manager.

McKee and colleagues note that the variability between clinical directorates shows the ability of doctors to adapt to managerial initiatives. More importantly, they emphasise the overwhelming sense of continuity rather than change, and 'few examples of trusts creating a new climate in which clinical directors of the future were being spotted, nurtured or sustained' (p. 110). Furthermore, clinical management was very thinly resourced, with many directorates run on a shoestring. The minority of directorates that were not traditionalist held out the prospect that clinicians could be developed into innovative leaders, but advocated for this to happen:

'more, and more senior, doctors will have to be given the incentive to get involved, the relevance of management will have to be actively marketed and the clinical legitimacy of doctor-managers will have to be safeguarded' (p. 112).

In many ways, this study reaffirmed evidence from the organisational theory literature relating to the tendency of professional bureaucracies to be oriented to stability rather than change, while also underlining the limited progress in moving from professional bureaucracies to managed professional businesses.

Further confirmation of the persistence of established relationships comes from Kitchener's study of the impact of quasi-market hospitals (Kitchener, 1999). Drawing on Mintzberg's writing (1979), Kitchener hypothesises that the NHS reforms are an attempt to replace the professional bureaucracy with the quasi-market hospital archetype. In this new archetype, the hospital is based around clinical directorates and medical cost centres, and a more businesslike approach to management is adopted, centred on medical cost centres and using enhanced management information systems. Kitchener found that in practice the impact of this new archetype was limited and warns that:

The fact that some hospital doctors have accepted medical-manager roles within a more integrated formal structure should not...be conflated with either a loss of their professional autonomy or a replacement of key elements of the PB (professional bureaucracy) interpretive scheme' (p. 197).

He concludes that the notion of the professional bureaucracy continues to provide an appropriate basis for understanding the nature of hospitals as organisations.

The challenges facing clinical directors were highlighted in a survey of doctor-manager relationships in Great Britain by Davies and colleagues. This survey found that senior managers such as chief executives and medical directors were more positive about these relationships than managers at directorate level. Among all the groups surveyed, clinical directors were the least impressed with management and the most dissatisfied with the role and influence of clinicians. Davies and colleagues argued that unless the divergence of views they found were addressed then it would be difficult to engage medical leaders in the government's modernisation agenda (Davies, Hodges, Rundall, 2003).

This conclusion echoes other work which concluded that clinical directors and other doctors in leadership roles occupied a 'no-man's-land' between the managerial and clinical communities (Marnoch, McKee, Dinnie, 2000). It is also consistent with the research of Degeling and colleagues (2003), which has described the differences that exist among staff groups in relation to individualist versus systematised conceptions of the financial and accountability aspects of clinical work. The existence of these differences confirms the persistence of tribal relationships in hospitals and the difficulties facing staff, such as doctors, who go into management roles and must bridge different cultures.

On a more positive note, one of the most comprehensive studies of medical managers noted evidence that clinical leaders can play an influential role as promoters of change. Fitzgerald and colleagues observed that, notwithstanding the proliferation of clinical director and medical director roles, and the establishment of BAMM as a professional association, clinical managers lacked a coherent identity and accepted knowledge base. They commented that:

'Externally, there is no recognition of clinical management as a specialty, with limited opportunities or credentials – and an unwillingness to undertake major training. Other medical professionals do not consider clinical management to represent a medical specialty – rather clinical mangers uncomfortably span the managerial/clinical divide and are not full or influential members of either occupational group' (Fitzgerald, Lilley, Ferlie, et al., 2006, p. 170).

In its work, BAMM reviewed the development of medical management roles in the NHS and set out a proposed career structure for medical managers such as medical directors, clinical directors and associate medical directors (BAMM, 2004). BAMM's proposals emphasised the need to properly reward and recognise the part played by medical management, and to make it an attractive career option for skilled and motivated doctors. These recommendations underline the need to link the development of medical leadership to appropriate incentives and career structures. As BAMM has argued:

> 'It is essential that medical management is rewarded and supported in a way that will attract the strongest applicants to the posts. Currently there are a number of major deterrents – for example the relative difficulties in describing and defining management activities. These activities can be more difficult to define as coherent sessions than is the case for clinical work. The lack of a clear concept of where a medical management career move will take the individual also proves to be a major barrier' (BAMM, 2004, p. 24).

Primary care was largely bypassed by the changes that flowed from the Griffiths Report, and only recently have there been moves to strengthen management and leadership in primary care. Work by Sheaff and colleagues (2003) has described the impact of these moves in primary care groups and trusts in England. Lacking any formal, hierarchical authority over GPs, primary care groups and trusts worked through GPs who took on the role of clinical governance leads, the Professional Executive Committee (PEC), medical directors and, more recently, practice-based commissioning lead roles. Medical leadership within primary care will become even more important if the coalition government's plan to introduce GP Commissioning Consortia and to devolve up to 80% of the NHS budget to them is implemented. Sheaff and his co-authors argue that clinical governance leads used a range of informal techniques to implement clinical governance in primary care, and they use the terms 'soft governance' and 'soft bureaucracy' to describe the relationships and organisations they studied.

In summary, research into medical leadership in the NHS since the Griffiths Report highlights the challenges involved in developing the role of medical managers. While progress has been made in appointing doctors as clinical directors and in establishing clinical directorates within hospitals, the effectiveness of these arrangements is variable. If in some organisations there appears to be much greater potential for involving doctors in leading change, in most there remain difficulties in changing established ways of doing things and in supporting medical leaders to play an effective part in bridging the divide between doctors and managers. Part of the explanation of these findings is the resourcing put into medical leadership and the limited recognition and rewards for doctors who take on leadership roles. Also important is the continuing influence of informal leaders and networks operating alongside formal management structures. Summarising the mixed experience of clinical directorates, Marnoch concluded his assessment in the following way:

> 'The means of controlling the operational performance of hospital doctors have advanced somewhat since the introduction of general management in the 1980s. Nevertheless, the Griffiths-inspired drive to push resource-consuming decisions down to the level where

they could best be made is far from complete. A traditional centralised style of manage-
ment has been used to make the internal market work. This form of control remains con-
strained in its influence over clinical behaviour. At worst, medical directors and clinical
directors will be used as go-betweens in a familiar book-balancing exercise that involves
closing wards periodically, not filling vacancies and cancelling operations. At best they
are the basis for a new strategically led style of corporate management in the NHS'
(Marnoch, 1996, p. 61).

MEDICAL LEADERSHIP: CRITICAL TO SERVICE TRANSFORMATION NATIONALLY AND LOCALLY

The NHS Plan (DH, 2000) was the culmination of three years of the Blair Labour
Government engaging with a wide variety of stakeholders, including the public. As
Ham (2004) suggests:

'. . . both the public and staff attached high priority to more and better paid staff. For
the public, reduced waiting times for treatment were important, while staff identified the
need for more training and "joined up working"' (p. 63).

A major element of the NHS plan was significantly greater investment, linked
to reforms based around redesign of care to improve access and stimulate higher
quality provision, i.e. continuous service improvement. Underlying these improvements was a strong performance regime with stringent, non-negotiable targets on,
for example, access, waiting times for consultants and treatments, cleanliness, financial control.

The NHS plan also introduced a new relationship between the Department of
Health and the NHS. This was clarified in *Shifting the Balance of Power* (DH, 2001),
which led to the establishment of strategic health authorities (initially 28, but subsequently reduced to 10), primary care trusts and the start of the movement to NHS
Foundation Trusts.

Whilst not as explicit on the importance of medical leadership and engagement
in implementing the reforms espoused in the NHS plan as perhaps Lord Darzi's
report in 2008, the former has clearly had a significant impact on changing the way
in which doctors contribute to the management, leadership and transformation of
services. However, the NHS Plan was unique in that the leaders of most of the major
medical professional bodies, along with many other national organisations including the British Medical Association, were co-signatories.

This national involvement and endorsement set a new tone around medical leadership and probably contributed to a new focus on doctors being more involved in
policy formulation at the national level. Slowly but surely it also acted as a trigger
for increasing engagement at the local level.

Yet, despite the stated intentions of the major reforms of the NHS in 1974, 1982
and the NHS Plan of 2000 of seeking to get doctors more involved in management,

there was no discernable change during the initial years of the 21st century. However, the tide began to turn around then as the movement around service and quality management began to gain momentum throughout the NHS.

Ham (2003) contends that it is particularly important to understand what motivates professionals. In Chapter 4 we refer to an evaluation study by Bowns and McNulty (1999) into the reengineering project at Leicester Royal Infirmary, which concluded that significant change in clinical domains cannot be achieved without the cooperation and support of clinicians.

A further study by McNulty and Ferlie (2002) showed that business process reengineering had variable impact in the hospital despite top management support. They concluded that consultants had the power to either promote or inhibit change.

Similar conclusions were reached by Ham and colleagues in a study on the implementation of the national booked admissions programme in 24 pilot sites. The study found substantial variation in progress between the sites. Some areas were more receptive to change than others, and the most successful pilots were those with a combination of a chief executive who made it clear that booking was a high priority for the organisation and medical champions who were willing to lead by example and exert peer pressure on reluctant colleagues (Ham *et al.*, 2003).

The NHS Modernisation Agency (2004) compiled a much applauded report – *10 High Impact Changes for Service Improvement and Delivery* – in 2004. This document suggested 10 changes that could be made across the NHS and achieve dramatic improvements in services:

> *'if these changes were adopted across the NHS to the standard already being achieved by some NHS organisations, there would be a quantum leap improvement in patient and staff experience, clinical outcome and service delivery – and waiting lists would become a thing of the past' (p. 8).*

It is clear that these evidence-based improvements have been demonstrated to have significant impacts on services through major initiatives such as the Improvement Partnership of Hospitals and the collaborative programmes. A number of these changes outline the importance of clinical leadership for their implementation. For example, one of the changes to increase day surgery rates was dependent on an identified clinical lead to effect the improved rates sought. Similarly, improving access to key diagnostic tests and a 'flow' of patients through the system required not only the use of service improvement methodologies and tools but also strong clinical leadership and the active engagement of clinical teams.

During the early years of the 21st century a new paradigm of medical leadership began to emerge. Built on the platform of the service improvement and modernisation movement, doctors began to see greater attraction in leading quality and safety improvements than they had hitherto in resource management. A number of general practitioners had become attracted to the opportunities afforded by influencing change through Fundholding and complex multi-funds in the early 1990s, which were reincarnated with far more rigour as commissioners through primary care groups initially, then subsequently primary care trusts and practice-based commissioning. This will be significantly enhanced by the Conservative-Liberal Democrat coalition government's plans to introduce GP Commissioning Consortia.

MEDICAL LEADERSHIP: THE PROFESSION REDEFINES ITSELF

In conjunction with the greater involvement of doctors in service improvement initiatives, it was clear that the nature of the profession of medicine was changing. Writing from an Australian perspective, Dowton (2004) indentified the traditional role of the medical profession as being defined through longstanding legislative canons coupled with the status accrued to individual doctors by society and societal contacts, and deeply entrenched cultural systems arising principally from the influence of professional craft groups. Dowton identified a number of external influences that have altered doctors' autonomy and the hierarchies within which they practise. He suggests that the influences include a greater demand for accountability for the safety of patients, quality and efficacy of healthcare and public access to medical information. Dowton concludes that, despite leadership roles being critical, inadequate attention has been paid to developing individual leaders and new models of leadership within the medical profession.

The Royal College of Physicians of London has made a significant contribution to the debate on the changing nature of the medical profession. *Doctors in society: medical professionalism in a changing world* (2005) contends that the medical profession is at a turning point in its history. The report argues that:

> *'Medicine bridges the gap between science and society. Indeed the application of scientific knowledge is a crucial aspect of clinical practice. Doctors are an important agent through which that scientific understanding is expressed. But medicine is more than that sum of our knowledge about disease. Medicine concerns the experience, feelings, and interpretation of human beings in extraordinary moments of fear, anxiety and doubt. In this extremely vulnerable position, it is medical professionalism that underpins the trust the public has in doctors' (p. 55).*

The College defines medical professionalism as a set of values, behaviours and relationships that underpin this trust. Under six main themes (leadership; teams; education; appraisal; careers and research), the report offers clear, practical recommendations that should lead not only to further improvements in patient care, but also offer more challenging and fulfilling lives for doctors. In particular it recommended strengthening leadership and managerial skills and identifying young doctors with the potential to move onto medical leadership roles. Perhaps the most important message in terms of medical management and leadership is the report's recommendation that:

> 'The complementary skills of leadership and "followership" need to be carefully documented and incorporated into a doctor's training to support professionalism. These skills argue strongly for managerial competence among doctors. An individual doctor's decisions have both clinical and managerial elements. There are signs that management skills will gradually become incorporated into fitness-to-practice requirements' (para 3.6).

Chapters 6 and 8 explore some of the international movements regarding medical leadership and the way in which, in particular, the CanMEDS framework developed by the Royal College of Physicians and Surgeons of Canada (2005) is influencing new definitions of 'a good doctor'.

Various influences have led to a marked change in the role of doctor in management, leadership and transformation of services on the last few years of the first decade of the 21st century. A new phenomenon has hit the NHS, with young doctors positively seeking to be involved and offered leadership development opportunities and senior medical leaders encouraging such diversions from specialty training. The journey recorded above has clearly had some impact. Why should there be such a dramatic twist in the medical leadership story now given all the previous initiatives?

Perhaps, the acknowledgement that there is a real correlation between medical engagement and leadership and quality outcomes is encouraging more doctors to not only move from the dark side but to centre stage. Leading service improvement appears to be far more attractive to doctors that the previous resource management representative roles. Furthermore, doctors in their clinical roles have historically been influenced by evidence. Perhaps, the increasing evidence of the relationship between medical leadership and engagement and quality of care is attracting more doctors to become involved.

In response to this dramatically changing environment, the NHS Institute for Innovation and Improvement and The Academy of Medical Royal Colleges developed a joint project to enhance the engagement of doctors in management, leadership and transformation of services. Established in early 2006, it is having a profound impact on the changing nature of the doctor in the 21st century. The joint King's Fund and Royal College of Physicians Report *Understanding Doctors: Harnessing professionalism* (2008) contends that:

> '. . . the world in which doctors work is changing, and changing in ways that challenge many of the assumptions on which the profession has based its practice for more than 150 years' (p. viii).

As Clark *et al.* (2008) contend, 'historically the medical profession in the UK has not particularly encouraged doctors to obtain competency in management and leadership. It has generally been left to individual doctors to voluntarily seek management and leadership training and development' (Clark *et al.*, 2008, p. 3). This is explored in more detail in Chapter 8.

This occurs despite the evidence that improving the health of the population and the delivery of high quality health and social care is very dependent on the support and active engagement of all doctors, not only in their practitioner activities but also in their management and leadership roles.

Whilst healthcare has always been complex, current societal demands have accentuated this. The NHS and other international health systems require skilled and competent doctors and other clinicians to deliver high-quality clinical care whilst working as part of a multidisciplinary team in an organisation or service designed to held staff to deliver safe and effective care. Medical training has traditionally focused on the clinical skills needed to be a safe and competent clinician. However, with the increasing trend to more team-based practice and integrated care approaches, it is important that doctors are not only competent clinicians but also have the skills to enable them to function effectively within these more complex systems. It is now recognised that to be a competent clinician requires doctors to be able to manage themselves and their time, work within a team, understand when to lead and when to follow, work in a more integrated way with other clinicians and services and deliver high quality and cost-effective best practice in a way that recognises the choices and preferences of patients.

The Final Report of the Independent Inquiry into Modernising Medical Careers (MMC Inquiry) supports this by contending that:

> 'The doctor's role as diagnostician and the handler of clinical uncertainty and ambiguity requires a profound educational base in science and evidence-based practice as well as research awareness. The doctor's frequent role as head of the healthcare team and commander of considerable clinical resource requires that greater attention is paid to managerial and leadership skills irrespective of specialism. An acknowledgement of the leadership role of medicine is increasingly evident. Role acknowledgement and aspiration to enhanced roles be they in subsequently practice, management and leadership, education or research are likely to facilitate greater clinical engagement. Encouraging enhanced roles will ensure maximum return, for the benefit society will derive from the investment in medical education' (MMC Inquiry, 2008, p. 17).

MEDICAL LEADERSHIP: AN ESSENTIAL INGREDIENT FOR SERVICE IMPROVEMENT

Thus, various initiatives, studies and reports in the middle of the first decade of the 21st century began to have considerable impact on the changing role of doctors and their involvement in the delivery of improved services.

It is perhaps not surprising that clinicians generally and doctors in particular were widely involved in the development of *High Quality Care for All: NHS Next Stage Review Final Report* (2008). As an eminent surgeon, Lord Darzi, its architect and author, had been appointed by Gordon Brown, Blair's successor as Prime Minister, in 2007 as a Parliamentary Under-Secretary of State (Health).

As with the NHS Plan, leading clinicians were co-signatories to *High Quality Care for All*. Whereas in the former, these were national leaders, Lord Darzi secured the support of the 10 Strategic Health Authority Clinical Leaders.

Darzi acknowledged that, whilst leading the Review, he had continued his clinical practice, reinforcing very publicly that combining clinical practice and leadership role was both feasible and perhaps to be positively encouraged.

Given his profession, it is perhaps not surprising that the new national and local clinical visions outlined in *High Quality Care for All* should have emerged from a wide number of local discussions involving over 2000 clinicians.

High Quality Care for All is far more explicit about the role of clinicians, particularly doctors, in leading service improvement, e.g.:

> *'what is clear is that this new professionalism, acknowledging clinician's roles as partners and leaders, gives them the opportunity to focus on improving not just the quality of care they provide as individuals but within their organisation and the whole NHS. We enable clinicians to be partners and leaders alongside manager colleagues' (para 5.7, p. 60).*

The need for greater clinical leadership is a common theme throughout *High Quality Care for All* (2008). However, it recognises that it is unrealistic to expect NHS staff to take on leadership without action to make it integral to training and development. The joint NHS Institute for Innovation and Improvement and Academy of Medical Royal Colleges initiative to develop a Medical Leadership Competency Framework for doctors at all stages of their training and careers, i.e. from undergraduate through postgraduate education to continuing practice has created a standard that can now be applied to all clinical professionals.

Prior to the publication of *High Quality Care for All* the Department of Health (England) appointed a Medical Director of the NHS for the first time. The role was conceived to give a stronger focus on medical leadership and engagement throughout the NHS. Since the publication of the Report, each of the 10 strategic health authorities has now appointed a full-time medical director to equally reinforce the importance of medical leadership and engagement at the local level.

The NHS Confederation has made a significant contribution to the debate on leadership generally and clinical leadership specifically in recent years. In acknowledging the emphasis on the leadership role of clinicians, particularly doctors, in *High Quality Care for All*, the NHS Confederation in its paper called the *Future of Leadership* (2009) welcomed the joint NHS Institute of Innovation and Improvement and Academy of Medical Royal Colleges initiative of integrating leadership into medical education. This is explored in more detail in Chapter 8.

The NHS Confederation paper also confirms that the Chief Executive of the NHS in England has repeatedly stated that he would like to see more chief executives from a medical background and specifically at least one doctor on each chief executive short list. As the Confederation argues,

'While being a doctor can bring important insights, so can being a nurse or an accountant. The real issue is that, if doctors are effectively excluded from chief executive positions, a major pool of talent is locked away from the system and we need all the talent that is available' (NHS Confederation, 2009, p. 4-5).

In Chapter 7 we explore in much more detail the strong evidence that exists on the relationship between engagement of doctors and organisational performance.

CONCLUSION

As this chapter has shown, the NHS has historically found it difficult to encourage doctors to take up medical leadership roles let alone chief executive positions. Whilst there are signs that this is changing and indeed there are a number of initiatives that are likely to support greater engagement, including appointment of full-time medical directors nationally and at each Strategic Health Authority with responsibility for promulgating medical leadership and engagement. Other initiatives such as the joint NHS Institute and Academy of Medical Royal Colleges project, the appointment of clinical fellows, and similar opportunities for young doctors to lead service improvement projects (and many more) are also contributing to the newly emerging culture of enhanced medical leadership and engagement. This will be explored in Chapter 9.

Monitor, the independent regulator of NHS Foundation Trusts, stresses the importance of clinicians having prominent roles in leadership, particularly in service-line management. In effect, service lines are the NHS Foundation Trust's equivalent of a commercial company's business unit. An increasing number of consultants are being motivated to take up leadership roles of service lines where genuine devolution of responsibility for an integrated set of clinical, operational and financial objectives and outcomes is offered.

Hitherto, doctors have been resistant to consider such opportunities, citing the need for clearer career paths both in and out of leadership roles, lack of proper leadership roles, lack of proper leadership training and preparation, reduced pay, job insecurity and loss of links with their profession. For many doctors the lack of access to clinical excellence awards have been cited as a further barrier, although the consultant contract does provide some flexibility, and amendments to the Clinical Excellence Awards Scheme are being introduced to reflect quality improvement and clinical leadership activities.

It is evident that many of these barriers are real, but others are perhaps more a perception of the culture which, with a few notable exceptions, has not positively encouraged doctors to make the leap into leadership roles.

The proposed introduction of the GP Commissioning Consortia will require highly effective leadership from many GPs. It is too early to assess the extent to which GPs generally will embrace the new leadership opportunities afforded by this new challenge and indeed whether individuals will have the necessary skills to realise the benefits sought from politicians. Nevertheless, it does confirm that the NHS is continuing its journey from a strong focus on general management to one increasingly based on medical leadership.

REFERENCES

Bate P. Changing the culture of a hospital: from hierarchy to networked community. *Public Administration.* 2000; **78**: 485–512.

Bowns IR, McNulty T. *Reengineering Leicester Royal Infirmary: an independent evaluation of implementation and impact.* Sheffield: School of Health and Related Research, University of Sheffield; 1999.

British Association of Medical Managers. *Making Sense – a career structure for medical management.* Stockport: The British Association of Medical Managers; 2004.

British Medical Journal. Doctors becoming managers: a conversation among Richard Smith, Sir Anthony Grabham and Professor Cyril Chantler [interview by Richard Smith]. *BMJ.* 1989; **298**(6669): 311–4.

Chantler C. Management reform in a London hospital. In: Carle N, editor. *Managing for Health Result.* London: King Edward's Hospital Fund for London; 1990.

Chantler C. Historical background: where have clinical directorates come from and what is their purpose? In: Hopkins A, editor. *The Role of Hospital Consultants in Clinical Directorates.* London: Royal College of Physicians; 1993.

Chantler C. *How to Treat Doctors: role of clinicians in management (speaking up: policy and change in the NHS).* NAHAT; 1994.

Clark J, Spurgeon P, Hamilton P. Medical Professionalism: leadership competency – an essential ingredient. *The International Journal of Clinical Leadership.* 2008; **16**(1): 3–9.

Davies HTO, Hodges C, Rundall T. Views of doctors and managers on the doctor-manager relationship in the NHS. *BMJ.* 2003; **326**: 626–8.

Degeling P, Maxwell S, Kennedy J, *et al.* Medicine, management and modernisation: a 'danse macabre'? *BMJ.* 2003; **326**: 649–52.

Department of Health. *The NHS Plan: a plan for investment, a plan for reform.* HMSO; 2000.

Department of Health. *Shifting the Balance of Power within the NHS: securing delivery.* London: Department of Health; 2001.

Department of Health. *High Quality Care for All: NHS Next Stage Review Final Report.* TSO; 2008.

Department of Health. *Equity and Excellence: liberating the NHS.* London: UK Stationery Office; 2010.

Dowton BS. Leadership in medicine: where are the leaders? *Medical Journal of Australia.* 2004; **181**(11–12): 652–4.

Fitzgerald L, Lilley C, Ferlie E, *et al. Managing Change and Role Enactment in the Professionalised Organisation.: report to the National Co-ordinating Centre for NHS Service Delivery and Organisation R&D.* London: NCCSDO; 2006.

Griffiths Report. *NHS Management Inquiry*. London: Department of Health and Social Security; 1983.

Ham C. Improving the performance of health services: the role of clinical leadership. *Lancet*. 2003; **361**(9373): 1978–80. Epub 25 March 2011.

Ham C. *Health Policy in Britain*. 5th ed. Basingstoke: Palgrave Macmillan; 2004.

Ham C, Kipping R, McLeod H. Redesigning work processes in healthcare: lessons from the National Health Service. *The Milbank Quarterly*. 2003; **81**: 415–39.

Hopkinson RB. Clinical Leadership in Practice – Wearing Many Hats, *Healthcare and Informatics Review Online*. 2004; **4**(9). Available at: www.hinz.org.nz/journal/498 (accessed 27 May 2011).

King's Fund and Royal College of Physicians. *Understanding Doctors: harnessing professionalism*. London: King's Fund; 2008.

Kitchener M. 'All fur coat and no knickers': contemporary organisational change in United Kingdom hospitals. In: Brock D, Powell M, Hinings C. *Restructuring the Professional Organisation*. London: Routledge; 1999.

Klein R. *The New Politics of the NHS*. 5th ed. Oxford: Radcliffe Publishing; 2006.

Levitt R, Wall A, Appleby J. *The Reorganised National Health Service*. 6th ed. Cheltenham: Stanley Thornes; 1999.

Marnoch G. *Doctors and Management in the National Health Service*. Buckingham: Open University Press; 1996.

Marnoch G, McKee L, Dinnie N. Between organisations and institutions. legitimacy and medical managers. *Public Administration*. 2000; **78**: 967–87.

McKee L, Marnoch G, Dinnie N. *Medical managers: puppetmasters or puppets? Sources of power and influence in clinical directorates*. In: Mark A, Dopson S, editors. *Organisational behaviour in healthcare: the research agenda*. Basingstoke: Macmillan; 1999.

McNulty T, Ferlie E. *Re-engineering Health Care: the complexities of organisational transformation*. Oxford: Oxford University Press; 2002.

Merivale SC. *Medical Organisation and Staffing in Modern Hospital Management*. The Institute of Hospital Administrators; 1969.

Ministry of Health. *Functions and constitution of medical staff committees*. R.H.B.(53)91/H.M.C.(53)85/B.G.(53)87; 1953.

Mintzberg H. *The Structuring of Organisations: a synthesis of the research*. Englewood Cliffs, NJ: Prentice Hall; 1979.

MMC Inquiry. *Aspiring to Excellence: final report of the independent enquiry into modernising medical careers*. London: Aldridge Press; 2008.

NHS Confederation. Developing NHS leadership: the role of the trust medical director. In: *Future of Leadership*. NHS Confederation; 2009. p. 2. Available at: www.nhsconfed.org/Publications/Documents/future_leadership020309.pdf (accessed 22 April 2011).

NHS Modernisation Agency. *10 High Impact Changes for Service Improvement and Delivery*. Department of Health; 2004.

Paton C, Whitney D, Cowpe J. Medical leadership: doctors, the state and prospects for improvement. In: Edmonstone J, editor. *Clinical Leadership: a book of readings*. Chichester: Kingsham Press; 2005.

Pollard M. On the side walk. *Health Service Journal*. 22–24 November 2001.

Rosenthal M. *The Incompetent Doctor: behind closed doors*. Buckingham: Open University Press; 1995.

Royal College of Physicians. Doctors in society: medical professionalism in a changing world. *Clin Med.* 2005 Nov–Dec; **5**(6 Suppl 1): S5–40.

Royal College of Physicians and Surgeons of Canada. *The CanMEDS Physician Competency Framework: better standards, better physicians, better care.* RCPSC; 2005.

Sheaff R, Rogers A, Pickard S, *et al.* A subtle governance: 'soft' medical leadership in English primary care. *Sociology of Health and Illness.* 2003; **25**(5): 408–28.

Simpson J. Clinical leadership in the UK. *Healthcare and Informatics Review Online.* 2004; 4(2). Available at: www.hinz.org.nz/journal/167 (accessed 27 May 2011).

Spurgeon P. Involving clinicians in management: a challenge of perspective. *Healthcare and Informatics Online.* 2001; 5(4). Available at: www.hinz.org.nz/journal/546 (accessed 27 May 2011).

Strong P, Robinson J. *The NHS Under New Management.* Milton Keynes: Open University Press; 1990.

An international overview: approaches to medical leadership in various systems

INTRODUCTION

The need to involve doctors in healthcare leadership has long been recognised (Berwick, 1994). Despite this, there is a perception in many healthcare systems that doctors are unhappy and in some cases alienated from the systems and organisations in which they work (Smith, 2001, and ensuing correspondence in the *BMJ*). The causes of doctors' unhappiness are many and varied, and are often imperfectly understood.

In their analysis, Edwards, Kornacki and Silversin (2002) hypothesise that part of the explanation is a breakdown in the implicit deal between doctors, patients, employers and society that defines what the parties to the relationship give and what they get in return. With doctors under increasing pressure to be accountable for their performance, deliver patient-centred care, and work collectively with other clinicians and staff to improve quality, Edwards and colleagues argue that the traditional psychological compact needs to be rewritten. One of the elements they propose should be in the new compact is the opportunity for doctors to shape the goals of their organisations and participate in resource allocation.

In the view of these authors, this requires a much bigger commitment to education and development for doctors to take on leadership and management roles, starting earlier in medical careers. The argument for supporting doctors to become more involved in leadership and management roles follows from the observation of:

> 'the crucial role that medical leaders (both formal and informal) play in setting the tone of the organisation and being a role model for others. This pivotal position as leaders, managers, and opinion formers in their organisations means that medical leaders at all levels have the opportunity to be instrumental in developing the dialogue about the 'gives' and 'gets' needed for a new compact' (Edwards, Kornacki, Silversin, 2002, p. 837).

Another reason for involving doctors in leadership is the evidence from research into quality improvement initiatives in healthcare that initiatives that fail to engage doctors tend to have a limited impact. At a time when issues of quality and patient safety are receiving increasing attention, medical leadership in raising standards and improving performance has been identified as a key priority for the future (Ham, 2003).

Further reinforcement of this insight comes from Mintzberg's analysis of healthcare organisations as professional bureaucracies rather than machine bureaucracies (Mintzberg, 1979). One of the characteristics of professional bureaucracies is that front-line staff members have a large measure of control by virtue of their training and specialist knowledge. Consequently, hierarchical directives issued by those nominally in control often have limited impact, and indeed may be resisted by front-line staff. Quality improvement in professional bureaucracies depends critically on the engagement of professionals and the ability of leaders who come from professional backgrounds to motivate their colleagues to change their behaviours and practices (Ham, Dickinson, 2008).

In this chapter we are interested in examining how doctors are involved in leadership roles within different health systems and indeed whether there are particular approaches to preparing doctors for the roles. As part of the Enhancing Engagement in Medical Leadership project conducted by the NHS Institute of Innovation and Improvement and the Academy of Royal Medical Colleges, a review of the approaches to preparing and involving doctors for leadership roles was commissioned. Experts in different countries were invited to prepare papers in their own systems and these were used to inform the framework for strengthening training and preparation for leadership roles developed by the NHS Institute and the Academy of Royal Medical Colleges. This chapter distils the key findings from the review (for the full report, *see* Ham, 2008) and focuses on the comparative context in which medical leadership is exercised. Other chapters discuss organisational and individual aspects of medical leadership in more detail.

REVIEW FINDINGS FROM AUSTRALASIA AND EUROPE

The papers prepared for the review covered experience in Australia, New Zealand, the Netherlands, Germany, Denmark, Finland, Norway and Sweden. Experts in these countries were invited in January 2007 to prepare papers describing the organisation and funding of the healthcare systems, the involvement of doctors in leadership roles in hospitals and in primary care, the education and development offered to doctors in leadership, and the content of leadership education and development. Draft papers were discussed at a workshop in May 2007, leading to the preparation of revised papers in July 2007. The findings were compared with the experience of the United Kingdom to inform the framework developed by the Academy of Medical Royal Colleges and the NHS Institute for Innovation and Improvement.

Subsequently, visits were undertaken to Canada and the United States to enable the experience of North America to be included in the work.

In all of the countries included in the review it was reported that it was unusual for chief executives of hospitals to come from medical backgrounds. Although some chief executives in all countries were doctors, it was much more common for senior doctors to take on the role of medical directors (or their equivalents) at board or senior management level. Within hospitals, doctors were also usually involved in leadership roles at the level of divisions, departments and directorates (the language varying between countries). These roles were analogous to the clinical director posts found in NHS hospitals, and typically involved the doctors concerned having a combined clinical and leadership role. Clinical directors of divisions and departments often worked as part of a team with support from general managers and/or nurse managers. In the case of Finland, Norway and Sweden, it was reported that there had been some weakening of the traditionally dominant role of doctors in leadership roles, driven by reforms that had strengthened the role of managers and challenged professional autonomy. This may help to explain the unhappiness of doctors in these countries.

Medical leadership in primary care appeared to be less well-developed than in hospitals in all countries. In large part, this was a consequence of the cottage industry nature of primary care provision and the lack of formal organisation compared with secondary care. With responsibility for primary care resting with doctors and their staff working within small teams and practices, the principal medical leadership roles involved doctors who were engaged in practice management and organising the business aspects of primary care provision such as contract negotiation, budget management and staffing. Only in countries such as New Zealand (through primary healthcare organisations) and England (through primary care trusts) have organisations been established to plan and manage primary care services. While doctors are involved in leadership roles in these organisations, as in hospitals this tends to be as medical directors or their equivalents rather than as chief executives. Compared with hospitals, medical work in primary care appears to be relatively unmanaged and reliant on traditional patterns of medical autonomy and self-regulation. This creates a major challenge in England, where the Conservative-Liberal Democrat coalition government that came to power in 2010 has acted quickly to reduce management costs and to set out proposals for general practitioners to lead the commissioning of health services.

Among all the systems studied, Denmark stood out as the country where there was an explicit aim of increasing the involvement of doctors in leadership roles. Mirroring experience in other countries, this was expressed in the appointment of medical directors to the boards of hospitals, with clinical departments within hospitals being required to have a medical leader. Of particular note in Denmark was the support provided to doctors to become leaders. At the postgraduate level, doctors received mandatory training in leadership based on demonstrating competences in seven roles derived from the CanMEDS approach developed in Canada (*see* Table 6.1). This included a 10-day leadership course provided by the Danish regions and the National Board of Health. After appointment as specialists, doctors were offered a five-day leadership course.

TABLE 6.1 The seven competences for Danish doctors*

1 The physician as *medical expert*

2 The physician *in collaboration*

3 The physician as a *communicator*

4 The physician as a *leader* and *administrator*

5 The *academic physician*

6 The physician as *promoter of health*

7 The *professional physician*

*This is developed in more detail in Chapter 8.

By comparison with Denmark, leadership education and development in other countries was less well-organised and was mainly offered to doctors following completion of their training on a voluntary basis when they were considering moving into leadership roles. To return to the analysis of Edwards, Kornacki and Silversin, there were no examples from the review of education and development starting earlier in doctors' careers, with undergraduate and postgraduate curricula dominated by scientific and clinical subjects.

The lack of systematic coverage of leadership as an area of study in the medical career pathway underlines the challenge of ensuring that doctors are equipped to meet leadership expectations as a normal and positive aspect of their roles.

EXPERIENCE IN NORTH AMERICA

As noted earlier, the findings of the review were supplemented by visits to Canada and the United States to gather information about experience in North America. In Canada, arrangements vary between provinces and also between hospitals. While it is unusual for hospital chief executives to come from medical backgrounds, this is more likely to be the case in the academic medical centres than in community hospitals. More commonly, regional health authorities and hospitals have a medical director, often known as the chief of staff or vice president of medical affairs, and this is often a full-time position. In addition, there are medical heads of divisions or departments who have a combined clinical and leadership role. The number of doctors in leadership roles varies between different types of hospitals, with small community hospitals tending to have the smallest number of medical leaders.

Doctors in Canada are not usually employed by hospitals but are independent physicians who have admitting rights and privileges and are paid on a fee-for-service basis. In some specialties this creates difficulties in recruiting doctors into leadership roles, not least because of the pay differential between clinical work and leadership positions. Leadership education and development is offered by individual hospitals, universities, health ministries and organisations such as the Canadian Medical Association (CMA). The Physician Manager Institute within the CMA provides a wide range of courses and programmes designed to increase medical leadership capacity (*see* www.cma.ca/index.cfm/ci_id/20291/la_id/1.htm). It is working with other organisations through the Canadian Health Leadership Network to strengthen healthcare leadership across Canada.

The position in the United States is more difficult to summarise accurately and succinctly because of the lack of an organised system of care in that country and the wide diversity of arrangements that exist. As in Canada, it is unusual for hospital chief executives to come from medical backgrounds, although a number of academic medical centres do have physician chief executives. Community hospitals usually have chief executives from non-medical backgrounds and place less emphasis on medical involvement in leadership. Another similarity with Canada is the key role played by the vice president of medical affairs, and the involvement of doctors as medical heads of divisions or departments. In the major academic medical centres such as New York Presbyterian, medical leaders are appointed jointly by the hospital leadership and the medical school, in recognition of the dual role they perform. The doctors who are appointed as chairs of departments take on prestigious roles within their organisations, and are often chosen through a highly competitive process, typically for a five-year, renewable term. One of the challenges in these organisations is balancing the academic and leadership credentials of departmental chairs.

Medical leadership education and development is offered by a wide range of organisations, including hospitals, universities, the Institute for Healthcare Improvement, and the American College of Physician Executives (*see* www.acpe.org/acpehome/index.aspx). The College offers an extensive programme of executive leadership development across the United States and is an important focus for community hospitals and other facilities that lack the resources to run their own in house activities. Some doctors supplement their medical training by obtaining qualifications in management and leadership. These qualifications include the Master of Public Health (management track), the Master of Business Administration (MBA), and the Master of Medical Management (MMM). In the case of the MBA, doctors in training may study for this concurrently, while in the case of the MMM, it is studied after the completion of medical training. In view of the diversity of arrangements in the United States, it is important to note that doctors who obtain qualifications in management and leadership may take on roles outside healthcare, e.g. in businesses associated with the healthcare industry, and do not always seek these qualifications because they wish to become leaders in hospitals or related organisations.

Although the provision of healthcare in the USA is difficult to capture in a general sense, there is emerging data supporting the critical role of doctors as leaders.

Of the 14 top hospitals/ health systems listed by US News and World Report as the best 5000 in the country, 11 are led by physicians. Similarly, over 50% of the best quality programmes are led by physicians.

Within the United States, Kaiser Permanente and Mayo Clinic are widely recognised as high-performing organisations that have given high priority to medical leadership. They were therefore selected for more detailed study.

KAISER PERMANENTE

Kaiser Permanente (KP) differs from most other forms of healthcare in the United States because it is an integrated system that provides almost all kinds of healthcare directly to its members. The main differences between the KP model and the non-integrated model are shown in Table 6.2. Established in the 1930s and opened to the public in 1945, KP comprises the Kaiser Foundation Health Plan, Kaiser Foundation Hospitals, and the Permanente Medical Groups. KP has expanded from its original home in California and currently comprises eight regions that serve members in nine states and the District of Columbia. As at the end of 2007, KP had 8.7 million members, operating revenues of around $38 billion and almost 160 000 employees. As well, the Permanente Medical Groups comprise 14 000 doctors who have a mutually exclusive relationship with the Kaiser Foundation Health Plan.

From the point of view of this book, it is the role of doctors in KP that is particularly interesting. The regionally based medical groups are partnerships or professional corporations of physicians which are self governing multispecialty physician organisations. Doctors become in effect shareholders in these groups after serving a period of probation or apprenticeship and being elected into membership by their

TABLE 6.2 Kaiser Permanente and the non-integrated model compared

KP model	Non-integrated model
Partnership of physicians and health plans	Competition between physicians and health plans
Mission-driven organisation: healthcare	Market-driven organisation: profit
Physicians cooperate and co-ordinate across specialties	Physicians practice in isolation from specialist colleagues
Non-profit health plan investments focussed on long-term quality and efficiency	For-profit health plan investments focussed on short-term stakeholder returns
Capitated prepayment encourages efficiency, prevention and wellness service	Fee-for-service payment encourages duplication, waste and over use of services
Partnering physicians help determine organisational strategies and priorities	Insurance executives/managers drive organisational strategies and priorities
Multidisciplinary, team-based care	Physicians practice in isolation

peers. The members of the medical groups in turn elect their leaders and hold them to account for their performance in a syndicalist-like arrangement.

The relationship of mutual exclusivity means that doctors only work with the Kaiser Foundation Health Plan and the Health Plan only contracts with doctors who are part of the Permanente medical groups. (The only exceptions to this relate to highly specialised care that cannot be provided within the medical group, and in areas where there are no Permanente physicians to serve Kaiser members. In these cases, the Health Plan will use contracted doctors.)

Permanente physicians are paid market rates, and some of their income is in the form of bonuses based on performance in areas like quality outcomes and patient experience. The remuneration package creates an incentive for doctors to stay within the groups, with pension entitlements being enhanced as retirement is reached. As a consequence, the fate of the medical groups and the plan is intertwined, and KP has found a way of aligning incentives to achieve and sustain high levels of performance in a competitive market.

Returning to Mintzberg's seminal analysis of the nature of healthcare organisations as the professional bureaucracies referred to earlier, a high proportion of doctors in these medical groups take on leadership roles. Roles include acting as physician-in-chief of a hospital or medical office, chief of a clinical department, and leadership of quality improvement and IT programmes. While the numbers of doctors in leadership roles varies between regions, it is not unusual for one quarter of physicians to be involved in some capacity, and in some parts of KP the proportion is closer to one-half. Doctors not in formal leadership roles are also involved in contributing to the work of the medical groups through participating in the development of drug formularies, clinical guidelines and related activities. The significance of this is that medical leadership is not an activity undertaken by a small proportion of the medical group but becomes part of the expectation of those working in the group and 'the way business is done around here'. Typically, medical leaders work closely with leaders from general management and nursing backgrounds in a medicine/management partnership (Crosson, 2003; *see also* Crosson, Weiland, Berenson, 2004).

It is within the medical groups that agreement is reached on how care should be delivered to members, with the emphasis being placed on achieving improvements in performance through the intrinsic commitment of doctors to do a good job rather than seeking their compliance with targets or standards set externally, although these also play a part. The result is a culture in which doctors take responsibility for performance and work with their peers to address areas of underperformance and achieve higher standards of care. Within this culture, extensive use is made of data on comparative performance. Medical leaders use these data to compare physicians and encourage changes in practice where these are needed. Peer comparison and peer pressure for improvement therefore lie at the heart of performance improvement, reflecting the importance attached to collegial processes and physician leadership in KP. This is reinforced by the use of financial incentives to reward good performance by physicians. While the incentives are not large, the experience of the medical groups is that physicians are naturally competitive, and even small amounts of additional income can act as positive stimulus to improvement.

The way of working found in KP has not emerged by accident. Rather, it reflects learning developed over many years, and the investment made in career-long education and professional development for doctors. This investment starts with the recruitment of new physicians and their induction into the medical group and continues as they gain experience and take on leadership roles of different kinds. The progression of doctors through these roles is planned as part of a career structure that enables physicians to undertake clinical and leadership responsibilities in different combinations as their career unfolds. Figure 6.1 illustrates in schematic terms the leadership development programme used in the Southern California Permanente Medical Group and the content of the curriculum used in the programme. Much of the education and development on offer is provided in-house through the specialist trainers and educators employed by the medical groups themselves, with additional support available from external organisations and experts. The involvement of all doctors in education and development contributes to the distinctive corporate culture found in KP and helps to promote followership as well as leadership among physicians.

There is stiff competition for posts within the medical groups, with many highly qualified applicants for each vacancy that is advertised. There is a degree of

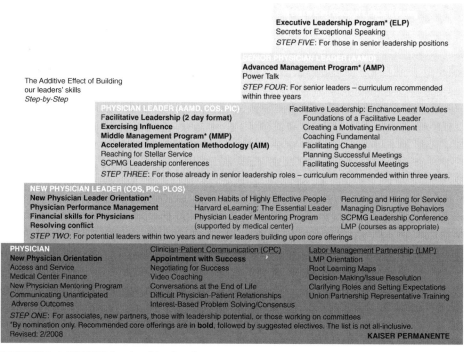

FIGURE 6.1 SCPMG leadership development

self-selection in this process, with doctors choosing to apply because of a preference for team working within an organised framework rather than competitive, office-based practice. The medical groups reinforce this preference through the education and development that is provided. Occasionally doctors do not find it easy to fit within the corporate culture. When this happens they may choose to leave, or the medical group may not invite them to continue practising following their three years on probation. More rarely, an established doctor may be asked to leave the group if there are concerns about performance that cannot be addressed within the group. Visitors from the UK are struck by the positive attitude of doctors in KP and the obvious pride they take in their work, and the organisation itself. In this sense, KP appears to be an exception to the universal tendency to unhappiness among doctors observed by Smith (2001) and others.

MAYO CLINIC

Mayo Clinic is the world's oldest and largest multispecialty group practice and is based in Rochester, Minnesota. It evolved from the medical practice of William Worrall Mayo, MD, an English doctor who emigrated to the United States in the 19th century. His sons, William James Mayo, MD, and Charles Horace Mayo, MD, took the family enterprise forward, incorporating other doctors and establishing a multispecialty practice. The Doctors Mayo worked closely with the Sisters of St. Francis, a Catholic teaching Order, in caring for the wounded survivors of a tornado that devastated Rochester in 1883.

From this experience, the Sisters founded Saint Marys Hospital in 1889 as an independent organization that worked closely with the outpatient practice of Mayo Clinic. The Sisters provided nursing care and administrative support, while the Mayos and their colleagues provided medical care. In 1919, the Mayo brothers converted their private practice into a not-for-profit organization, which has continuously evolved as an integrated delivery system. Saint Marys Hospital and its counterpart, Rochester Methodist Hospital, became part of Mayo's corporate structure in 1986. Today, Mayo Clinic is a world-renowned specialist centre of excellence that employs around 50 000 staff and has expanded beyond Minnesota to provide care in Arizona and Florida (for a recent analysis, *see* Berry, Seltman, 2008).

The origins of Mayo Clinic are of more than historical interest. Visitors are struck by the emphasis still placed on the values and principles of the Mayo family – particularly the brothers who built on their father's ideas. Mayo Clinic's primary value is that 'The needs of the patient come first'. This includes having time for patients, listening to them, ensuring their care is co-ordinated, and striving to achieve the best possible outcomes.

Mayo Clinic's symbol is three overlapping shields. These represent patient care, research and education. The mission of Mayo Clinic is to 'provide the best care to every patient every day through integrated clinical practice, education and research'.

In pursuing its mission, Mayo Clinic distinguishes itself from other integrated systems (for example, KP) that do not have the same combination of patient care, research and education. It also distinguishes itself from academic medical centres through the emphasis placed on the primary value of patient-centred care.

Mayo Clinic describes itself as 'physician led and administratively managed'. As in KP, physicians are salaried and have a relationship of mutual exclusivity with the Clinic. They are involved in leadership roles right through the organisation. Several aspects of physician leadership in Mayo are noteworthy. These include the following:

- physicians serve as departmental chairs, chairs of divisions within departments, chairs of the many committees that exist, and members of other committees. They serve as chief executive officers of the different sites (Rochester, Florida and Arizona) and of the enterprise as a whole. They lead education, research and clinical practice. They also lead the work of teams at the microsystem level
- physician leaders serve for limited terms, and the expectation is that they will move on at the end of their terms, e.g. a departmental chair typically serves for 8–10 years. Physicians move into senior leadership roles having gained experience in more junior roles. Physician leaders combine clinical and leadership responsibilities to facilitate their return to full-time clinical work at the appropriate time
- physician leadership roles are valued in the organisation and are for the most part sought after. There will usually be two or three candidates for the departmental chair roles when these become vacant. Physician leadership roles are invariably filled internally. There is an extensive process of consultation and debate with staff to ensure the right appointments are made (though sometimes mistakes happen)
- Mayo Clinic's culture downplays the roles of individuals and discourages the emergence of 'stars'. Instead, the emphasis is placed on teamwork (going back to the founding values), and conformity with Mayo Clinic's way of doing business ('everyone is dispensable'). As a result, there is a tendency to favour 'reluctant leaders' over those who are outwardly ambitious. The European history/origins (Scandinavia as well as England) are important here
- physician leaders receive a small salary supplement, but this is not significant and not the main motivator for those taking on leadership roles
- one of the challenges is the transition of physicians from leadership roles to clinical work. There is a sense that this could be done better and a task force has been established to come up with ideas for improvement.

Physician leaders at every level work in partnership with administrators. This is the meaning of 'physician led and administratively managed', and goes back to the early days of Mayo Clinic. There is mutual respect between physicians and administrators that facilitates partnership working.

In the last decade, increasing importance has been attached to training and development to support physicians to take on leadership roles. This is usually provided within Mayo Clinic, and the content of the programmes that are delivered is based on a four-part curriculum. The curriculum encompasses newly appointed staff, newly appointed leaders and their teams, experienced leaders, and senior leadership. Key competences have been identified for physician leaders. These are personal attributes, people leadership, business acumen and strategic leadership. Coaching and mentoring are offered as appropriate. Because of the emphasis on partnership between physicians and administrators, the number of physicians who have MBAs, MMMs and similar qualifications is low because administrators bring this expertise to the relationship. Mayo Clinic puts great effort into developing strong administration as well as physician leadership. It recruits graduates into its own management training scheme as well as hiring in the market, with more senior administrators coming up through the ranks rather than being recruited from the outside.

As in KP, a large proportion of physicians is in or has been in leadership roles. The system of term limits and rotating leadership is seen to facilitate this by ensuring regular turnover and also enabling the development of followership. This is because physicians often have experience in the challenges of leading relatively autonomous professionals, and are therefore more willing to support colleagues who are leaders. There is a sense in the organisation that 'everyone is a leader'. Underpinning these characteristics is a system of hiring staff that focuses on picking the best but also ensuring a good fit with Mayo Clinic's culture. This is helped by Mayo Clinic having a significant role in education, including running its own medical school and residency programme. Many physicians work their way up through training to become associate consultants. They serve for three years in this role 'on probation' before being confirmed as full consultants. During this time the expectation is that physicians who do not fit Mayo Clinic's culture will move out, i.e. there will be a cull. Once appointed, they tend to stay throughout their careers, and annual turnover is tiny (2–3%, including retirements).

Mayo Clinic's salaries relate to the market but are more closely aligned with market rates for some specialists than others. Physicians who want to make lots of money do not join Mayo Clinic. Despite this, Mayo Clinic attracts high-calibre physicians who have a preference for teamwork and working within an organised and integrated system (this includes having a well-developed IT system and electronic medical record). Mayo Clinic appeals to the intrinsic motivation of doctors to do a good job rather than providing financial incentives. With incentives playing a small role, alignment is achieved through physician leadership and organisational culture. The culture is sustained through continual reference to the founding values and principles and through orientation and ongoing development of physicians and other staff.

One important feature is the extensive use made of committees to work through issues with a perception that 'Mayo is a committee driven organisation'. This has strengths in ensuring widespread debate and deliberation, and ultimately buy-in when decisions are made. It also has weaknesses in being slow and sometimes frustrating for those involved. But again it is entrenched in the culture and an important aspect of how work gets done.

CONCLUSION

The results of the review summarised here highlight similarities and differences in the involvement of doctors in leadership in the countries studied. Among the countries covered in the survey of international experience, Denmark appears to have made most progress in supporting doctors to take on leadership roles, while Kaiser Permanente and Mayo Clinic are exemplars of organisations in which doctors play a major part in leadership and performance improvement. The broader lesson from the experience of KP and Mayo Clinic is that involving doctors in leadership requires that attention be paid to a range of factors, including:

- education and development at induction and throughout their careers in the skills needed to be effective team players, leaders and followers, etc.
- the career structures that enable doctors to move into and out of leadership roles, and to combine leadership and clinical responsibilities
- the value placed on medical leadership roles, not only in terms of financial reward but also in how the organisation sees these roles and recognises the individuals who take them on
- the proportion of physicians involved in leadership roles to enable participation in leadership to become part of the expectation of doctors rather than a minority interest
- an organisational culture that creates an expectation that physicians will take on leadership roles and that other physicians will serve as effective followers.

It is this package of factors that is likely to be critical in strengthening medical leadership, not simply ensuring that chief executives and other senior managers come from medical backgrounds, or indeed that education and development are strengthened to support doctors to take on leadership roles.

As far as education and development are concerned, much remains to be done to embed understanding of leadership issues throughout the training of doctors, starting during time spent at medical school. In this regard, the work being done by the Academy of Medical Royal Colleges and the NHS Institute for Innovation and Improvement to develop the Medical Leadership Competency Framework and to apply the framework at different stages in the career of doctors may enable the NHS to leapfrog systems that are further ahead, like Denmark, and position the UK at the forefront of international developments in this field. In reality, this will only happen in practice if the investment now being made in education and development is matched by a focus on the other factors identified above, including the career structures available to doctors, the value placed on medical leadership roles, and increasing the proportion of doctors involved in leadership.

ACKNOWLEDGEMENT

Chapter 6 is based on a paper previously published in *The International Journal of Clinical Leadership* (2008; **16**: 11–16).

REFERENCES

Berry L, Seltman K. *Management Lessons from Mayo Clinic*. New York, NY: McGraw-Hill; 2008.

Berwick D. Eleven worthy aims of clinical leadership of health system reform. *JAMA*. 1994; **272**(1): 792–802.

Crosson F. Kaiser Permanente: a propensity for partnership. *BMJ*. 2003; **326**: 654.

Crosson F, Weiland A, Berenson R. Physician leadership: 'group responsibility' as key to accountability in medicine. In: Enthoven A, Tollen L, editors. *Toward a 21st Century Health System: the contributions and promise of prepaid group practice*. San Francisco, CA: Jossey-Bass; 2004.

Edwards N, Kornacki M, Silversin J. Unhappy doctors: what are the causes and what can be done? *BMJ*. 2002; **324**: 835–8.

Ham C. Improving the performance of health services: the role of clinical leadership. *Lancet*. 2003; **361**(9373): 1978–80.

Ham C, editor. *Enhancing Engagement in Medical Leadership: a rapid survey of international experience*. Coventry: NHS Institute for Innovation and Improvement Academy of Medical Royal Colleges and Health Services Management Centre, University of Birmingham; 2008.

Ham C, Dickinson H. *Engaging Doctors in Leadership: what can we learn from international experience and research evidence?* Coventry: NHS Institute for Innovation and Improvement, Academy of Medical Royal Colleges and Health Services Management Centre, University of Birmingham; 2008. Available at: www.institute. nhs.uk/images/documents/BuildingCapability/Medical_Leadership/Engaging%20 Doctors%20in%20Leadership%20What%20we%20can%20learn%20from%20 international%20experience%20and%20research%20evidence.pdf (accessed 23 April 2011).

Mintzberg H. *The Structuring of Organisations*. Englewood Cliffs: Prentice-Hall; 1979.

Smith R. Why are doctors so unhappy? *BMJ*. 2001; **322**: 1073–4.

US News and World Report. *Best Hospitals 201–11: The Honor Role*. Available at: http:// health.usnews.com (accessed 23 April 2011).

CHAPTER 7

Why does it matter? Medical engagement and organisational performance

INTRODUCTION

Earlier chapters have illustrated the vital role of leadership, and in particular, medical leadership in the process of creating sustained system reform. Ham (2003) summarises key aspects of this context of change. He points to the distance between policy initiatives whether managed competition or integrated care and the day-to-day delivery of care by health professionals. Over the past 30 years, the NHS in the UK has acquired an unenviable reputation for the frequency with which it undertakes organisational restructuring. The cynicism of many doctors has been fuelled by their observation of this process and the contrasting reality of their own practice, where they will typically say: patients just keep turning up whatever politicians do with the system. It is surely the direct experience of patients in receiving treatment and the outcomes achieved that represent the true focus of system reform.

Policymakers must therefore, in designing changes or reforms, recognise that in order to be implemented successfully, the impact on patients must be apparent to those who have to enact the new system. Consultation with and involvement of clinical staff is therefore crucial to system reform. However, there is, as Ham points out, a reciprocal requirement on doctors in particular to recognise that politicians represent the public and that their attempts at reform (whether sound or not) are often well-intentioned attempts to achieve improvements for the user, the patient. Inevitably, some system changes will impinge upon the work of front-line staff, notably the setting of targets and formulation of priorities. At times, such policy initiatives have been resented by doctors as limitations upon their autonomy and professional discretion in the discharge of their practice. However, society has changed dramatically in terms of levels of education, accountability and the relative power of professional elites. Political initiatives empowering the public/patient and the erosion of traditional medical power bases is a manifestation of this change. There are many levels at which the processes of change may operate: Chapter 4 has made the case for the importance of clinical leadership in undertaking reform at a system-wide level. Though for the majority of health professionals and indeed for patients it is at the organisational level that the impact of change seems most real. The role of clinical leadership at this organisational level needs to be demonstrated, and the remainder of this chapter will explore some of the inter-related concepts of performance, leadership and engagement.

ORGANISATIONAL PERFORMANCE

There can be no doubt that healthcare providers have come under increasing scrutiny in the last two decades. Greater accountability through centrally defined targets has been a major focus of health policy, certainly in the UK. It would seem then that at face value it should be possible to assess how organisational performance, as measured by defined targets, is linked to good medical leadership. In fact, the evidence is relatively thin. In part this is due to a lack of clarity around what we mean by medical leadership, or even leadership per se, and how it might be assessed as good, bad or indifferent. High-profile cases such as in Mid-Staffordshire NHS Foundation Trust point to failures of medical leadership but more sophisticated analysis is needed to understand the attributional link between organisational performance and medical leadership.

Smith (2005) presents a fairly persuasive argument that suggests the way in which performance management through targets has not really facilitated the link to medical leadership. He argues that almost all the performance indicators have been directed explicitly or implicitly at the managerial community. The high level at which indicators have been defined has in his view been aimed at focusing 'the attention of senior managers of NHS organisations on government priorities, in what might be thought of as a form of "executive accountability"'. A great weakness of the traditional performance culture is its failure to engage the health professions. This also represents the greatest opportunity for a new focus in the way in which a more creative, innovative and clinically oriented performance culture could be developed. The Next Stage Review conducted by Lord Darzi illustrates this perfectly with its core theme of shifting the emphasis of performance parameters to service quality (Darzi, 2008).

This rather critical perspective on the use of performance indicators was strengthened further by Hauck *et al.* (2003), who suggested that there was a severe limitation on the degree to which managers could actually influence certain outcome measures. A similarly themed and influential paper by Mannion *et al.* (2005) suggested that star ratings of acute hospitals (the favoured system at the time) could produce a range of unintended and dysfunctional consequences, notably a limited, tunnel vision and distortion of clinical priorities; bullying and intimidation of staff; and a sapping of confidence for staff and the public.

Notwithstanding concerns about the nature of performance management and its implications, there is a growing body of evidence suggesting that good management practice and effective leadership can have a positive impact on organisational performance.

LEADERSHIP AND PERFORMANCE

West *et al.* (2002) focused particularly on people management and what might be called human resource management. An index of good human resource management practices was found to relate significantly to patient mortality in a sample of acute hospitals. The conduct of good appraisal and training systems was identified as being of particular importance. The paper makes a persuasive argument for the role of appraisal describing the process as 'directing employee performance towards achieving organisational goals and to improve individual performance' (p. 1308).

The data is consistent with findings in the private sector. The establishment of good appraisal systems with good levels of coverage and follow-up action may well be part of a well-run organisation. It is a little less clear how the link between appraisal of medical staff, which was relatively new to this staff group (and hence variable in coverage and focus) and specific clinical outcome measures like death after emergency surgery might be operating in an attributional model. Nonetheless the study has stimulated many attempts to explore the causal linkage more specifically, and in particular how leadership may relate to performance.

The difficulty of obtaining clear evidence of attribution between leadership and organisational performance is well-illustrated by Sutherland and Dodd (2008) in a description of their study evaluating the impact of a major leadership development initiative on clinical practice. In many ways it was an exemplary qualitative study, reporting many statements of perceived benefits from participants such as greater self-awareness, self-confidence and a more positive perspective on problem solving. However, it failed to identify any particular organisational benefits or specific changes to clinical practice. They conclude that this supports the assertion (Edmonstone, Western 2002) that there is no established consensus on what organisational benefits might be anticipated from leadership development programmes.

Keroack *et al.* (2007) took a different approach in attempting to determine what features of leadership might relate to high-performing academic medical centres. They identified key factors such as leaders with an authentic, hands-on style able to relate day-to-day events to the overall goal and a strong alliance between executive leadership and the clinical department chairs: Shipton *et al.* (2008) set out to examine the mechanisms by which leadership influences performance. It should be noted that the nature and level of leadership was assessed through staff perceptions of leadership. The findings suggest significant relationships between perceived leadership effectiveness and Commission for Health Improvement Star Ratings and with patient complaints. As the authors acknowledge, attribution of causality is not certain. Regardless the paper concludes that 'effective leaders shape organisational outcomes through creating a vision and building the allegiance of individuals and teams' (p. 443). Chapter 3 explores the various approaches and models of leadership in more depth, but it is probably true to say most discussions of leadership and organisational performance relate to non-medical managers. The literature focuses upon executives from many backgrounds and many sectors. In the context of this chapter it is perhaps Shipton *et al.*'s use of the term 'allegiance' that offers a route into the notion of engagement. Doctors, as we have seen, have a very strong allegiance to their professional bodies but not always so clearly with the organisation and its wider goals. Engagement may be the concept that can bring together individual professional identity within a more corporate context.

MEDICAL ENGAGEMENT: EXPLORING THE CONCEPT

Engagement has become a popular, much used term supplanting more traditional concepts such as job satisfaction and motivation. As is often the case with words that acquire a currency of usage they are often misused, losing specific meaning and acquiring a catch-all status. Politicians often link engagement to an area of conflict, claiming that we must engage the public in a debate about this issue. This presents engagement as a sort of event. It is not clear where, when or how this debate actually takes place but it is somehow happening, probably in forms of the media. This is probably to use the term engagement more as a form of consultation. Others use engagement as a solution, a general 'good thing', and that after engagement has happened there will be progress. In any event there is virtually never any attempt at definition or reference to where the term has come from and what people who use it actually mean by it.

Freeney and Tiernan (2006) provide a helpful overview of the literature on the emergence and development of the concept of engagement. Kahn (1990) argued that 'people can use varying degrees of their selves physically, cognitively and emotionally, in work role performances' (p. 670). Kahn also defined a state of disengagement and this was akin to Maslach and Jackson's (1986) concept of burnout, where the employee withdraws from the work role. The approach to engagement incorporating the notion of burnout rather emphasises a dimensional concept of burnout at one end and engagement at the other. This is probably an oversimplification, and subsequently engagement began to be defined as a separate construct in its own right.

Schaufeli and Bakker (2003) describe engagement as 'a persistent, positive affective motivational state of fulfilment in employees that is characterised by vigour, dedication and absorption' (p. 22). It is the differentiation of engagement into sub-components that is critical to attempts to identify relative strengths and weaknesses in terms of levels of engagement and to posit potential interventions that may promote higher levels. The current approach reported later in this chapter builds directly upon this notion.

The essential hypothesis of the engagement model is that higher levels of engagement generate a greater frequency of positive affect, such as satisfaction and commitment, and this in turn flows through to enhanced work performance. It is clearly a multifaceted concept, and some aspects of directionality, i.e. which aspects cause what in different circumstances and in different individuals, may be difficult to pin down. However, research has sought to explore the key aspects of what causes higher levels of engagement and what might be the consequences (outcomes) for the organisation of achieving higher levels of engagement.

Harter *et al.* (2003) report that employee engagement was associated with a range of business outcomes, such as higher levels of performance (.38), customer satisfaction and loyalty (.33) and lower levels of staff turnover (−.30). Although significant, Freeney and Tiernan (2006) suggest the results be treated with caution, as correlations are relatively small. Nonetheless, Salanova *et al.* (2005) describe improved customer satisfaction in the service sector relating to enhanced engagement, and Bernthal (2003) summarises research conducted by the Center for Applied Behavioral Research within Development Dimensions International that suggests similarly that when engagement scores are high employees are more satisfied, less likely to leave the organisation and more productive.

In the context of healthcare, Guthrie (2005) argues that physician engagement is one of the key priorities for chief executives and that success in this is one of the markers of better-performing hospitals. He argues that at a structural level (creating appropriate facilitative arrangements) and a personal level (one-to-one communication), it is possible for executives and managers to build up levels of physician engagement. Toto (2005), using Gallup survey data, demonstrates that engaged physicians can have a direct day-to-day impact on the financial bottom line of hospitals. The relationship between doctors and hospitals in the USA is rather different from that in the UK and other countries where more direct employment by the healthcare organisation is the norm. In Toto's study the continued use of and admitting preferences by independent doctors clearly impacts upon the hospital's income in a more direct business model arrangement. Engagement of physicians in Toto's study is manifest through aspects such as confidence in the hospital to deliver the services promised, a belief (integrity) that the hospital treats patients fairly and a pride and passion about being linked to a high-quality care provider.

A recent overview report by Macleod and Clarke (2009) provides an excellent account of employee engagement in the UK and in a range of sectors. In the report they reiterate, as in this chapter, that the term engagement has acquired a range of meanings and that no universal definition exists. However, despite this they make some important assertions about the concept:

- that engagement is a two-way process involving organisations working to engage employees and the latter having a degree of choice as to their response
- that engagement is measurable – with some variability in the evidence gained by different measurement tools
- that engagement correlates with performance and with innovation. Whilst recognising that proving direct causal links are important, the report concludes

that the consistent nature of the studies of engagement coupled with individual company case studies makes for a 'compelling case'

- engagement levels in the UK are relatively low, and this presents a major challenge given the critical nature of innovation in tackling the recession.

Macleod and Clarke (2009) provide many examples of reports and case studies from organisations where levels of engagement or attempts to promote engagement appear to relate to enhanced performance. It should be noted (as Macleod and Clarke acknowledge) that they have not been able to validate all the studies quoted. Many use internal survey instruments with slightly variable ways of assessing engagement, and there is rarely any mention of control or comparison groups so one cannot be entirely sure that a classic 'Hawthorn' effect is not at play. However, a meta-analysis of a series of Gallup studies by Harter *et al.* (2006) found consistently that business units in the top half of the engagement scores had 27% higher profitability than those in the bottom half. Similarly, engagement levels seemed to predict sickness absence, with more engaged employees taking 2.7 days per year compared to 6.2 days for disengaged employees.

Alimo-Metcalfe and Bradley (2008) exploring types of leadership in mental health teams in the NHS report that only 'engaging with others' was a significant predictor of performance. It is not only the organisation that seems to benefit from higher levels of engagement. So too does the individual member of the organisation with several accounts of a greater sense of well-being, more positive feelings about work and lower levels of mental health problems, e.g. anxiety and depression (Black, 2008; Waddell, Burton, 2006).

The evidence then would seem to be very powerful that engagement is a crucially important concept in promoting both individual well-being and organisational success. As Macleod and Clarke (2009) conclude from their review, the role of the leader (or leaders) in developing engagement is vital, but many leaders do not possess, or perhaps do not even value some of the 'soft' skills that may be necessary. Enhancing engagement is going to demand different and more subtle skills of leadership.

APPROACHES TO MEASURING AND DEVELOPING ENGAGEMENT FOR ORGANISATIONAL PERFORMANCE

As Ham and Dickenson (2008) comment in their review of medical leadership, engagement and organisational performance, very few measures of engagement are to be found that meet robust psychometric criteria. A major contribution though is that of Reinertsen *et al.* (2007) and colleagues from the Institute for Healthcare Improvement (IHI). Given the evidence supporting the importance of engagement they express surprise at how few hospitals have 'actually articulated a plan to improve the engagement of their physicians' (p. 2). Based upon working with and close observation of high-performing hospitals, they offer a framework for how organisations might go about improving levels of engagement. The basic framework is as follows:

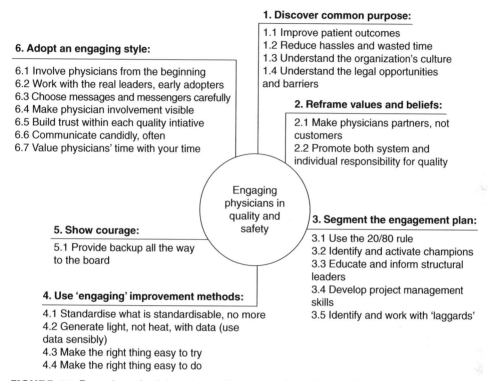

1. Discover common purpose:
1.1 Improve patient outcomes
1.2 Reduce hassles and wasted time
1.3 Understand the organization's culture
1.4 Understand the legal opportunities and barriers

6. Adopt an engaging style:
6.1 Involve physicians from the beginning
6.2 Work with the real leaders, early adopters
6.3 Choose messages and messengers carefully
6.4 Make physician involvement visible
6.5 Build trust within each quality intiative
6.6 Communicate candidly, often
6.7 Value physicians' time with your time

2. Reframe values and beliefs:
2.1 Make physicians partners, not customers
2.2 Promote both system and individual responsibility for quality

Engaging physicians in quality and safety

5. Show courage:
5.1 Provide backup all the way to the board

3. Segment the engagement plan:
3.1 Use the 20/80 rule
3.2 Identify and activate champions
3.3 Educate and inform structural leaders
3.4 Develop project management skills
3.5 Identify and work with 'laggards'

4. Use 'engaging' improvement methods:
4.1 Standardise what is standardisable, no more
4.2 Generate light, not heat, with data (use data sensibly)
4.3 Make the right thing easy to try
4.4 Make the right thing easy to do

FIGURE 7.1 Engaging physicians in quality and safety. *Source:* Reinersten JL, Gosfield AG, RuppW, *et al. Engaging Physicians in a Shared Quality Agenda* [IHI Innovation Services White Paper]. Cambridge, MA: 2007; 4. Available at: www.IHI.org (accessed 27 May 2011).

Each of these areas needs to be placed in the organisation's own context, and inevitably one or two operate in a US health system more directly than in the UK, but the principles are sound. An associated checklist presents organisations with the opportunity of rating themselves in terms of key areas of functioning (seven items with a maximum score of seven). Depending upon the score obtained, the Framework then describes some actions organisations can take to improve engagement. The standing of IHI has led to the Framework being quite influential in the area, but as a measure of engagement it is quite limited even though it works well in stimulating a dialogue and potential action to improve engagement.

It was in this general context – strong support for the concept of medical leadership and engagement as critical to performance, but deficiencies in terms of existing measures of engagement, that the joint Institute for Innovation and Improvement and Academy of Medical Royal Colleges Enhancing Engagement in Medical Leadership project set out to address the issue of medical engagement and organisational performance.

The measures of engagement that do exist tend to focus upon the feelings of individual staff and do not simultaneously evaluate the associated cultural conditions of the organisation. Moreover, no assessment tool exists that is designed to focus upon medical engagement – the specific context for the Enhancing Engagement in Medical Leadership project. There were three specific aims:

- to develop a reliable and valid measure of medical engagement that will be quick and relatively unobtrusive to complete
- to differentiate within the scale and measure of personal engagement at an individual level (the motivation of the individual to perform in appropriate managerial and leadership roles) from the organisational context (which may foster or constrain engagement)
- to develop a systematic framework for recommending organisational strategies for enhancing medical engagement and performance at work.

These goals and the process of development were based on three conceptual premises:

I   medical engagement is critical to implementing many of the radical changes and improvements sought in the NHS, and engagement levels are not universally high

II medical engagement cannot be understood from consideration of the individual employee alone. Organisational systems play a crucial role in providing the cultural conditions under which the individual's propensity to engage is either encouraged or inhibited. The measure must therefore simultaneously assess both the individual and cultural components of the engagement equation and this is reflected in the operational definition of engagement used in the development process. The active and positive contribution of doctors within their normal working roles to maintaining and enhancing the performance of the organisation which itself recognises this commitment in supporting and encouraging high quality care

III a distinction is made between competence and performance in the context of work behaviour. Competence may be thought of as what an individual can do, but this is not the same as what they will do the two together equalling performance.

PROCESS OF DEVELOPMENT

Applied Research Ltd. (a relatively small research and consultancy organisation) had previously developed a Professional Engagement Scale, with data on over

23,000 healthcare professionals. In the timescale of the overall project it was felt that an adaptation of this existing scale to medical engagement was the most effective route. This involved refining the existing scale items to provide a medical engagement focus, piloting the items with an appropriate population and then undertaking relevant psychometric analysis to confirm the reliability and validity of the scales.

The re-analysis of the original data-set (23 782 NHS staff) using factor analysis produced a hierarchical scale structure as presented below:

MES Scale	Scale definition (The scale is concerned with the extent to which ...)
Index: Medical engagement	... doctors adopt a broad organisational perspective with respect to their clinical responsibilities and accountability
Meta Scale 1: Working in an open culture	... doctors have opportunities to authentically discuss issues and problems at work with all staff groups in an open and honest way
Meta Scale 2: Having purpose and direction	... medical staff share a sense of common purpose and agreed direction with others at work particularly with respect to planning, designing and delivering services
Meta Scale 3: Feeling valued and empowered	... doctors feel that their contribution is properly appreciated and valued by the organisation and not taken for granted
Sub Scale 1: [O] Climate for positive learning	... the working climate for doctors is supportive and one in which problems are solved by sharing ideas and joint learning
Sub Scale 2: [I] Good interpersonal relationships	... all staff are friendly towards doctors and are sympathetic to their workload and work priorities
Sub Scale 3: [O] Appraisal and rewards effectively aligned	... doctors consider that their work is aligned to the wider organisational goals and mission
Sub Scale 4: [I] Participation in decision-making and change	... doctors consider that they are able to make a positive impact through decision-making about future developments
Sub Scale 5: [O] Development orientation	... doctors feel that they are encouraged to develop their skills and progress their career
Sub Scale 6: [I] Commitment and work satisfaction	... doctors feel satisfied with their working conditions and feel a real sense of attachment and commitment to the organisation

Here we can see the overall Index of Medical Engagement made up of a series of sub-scales:

- Meta Scale 1 Working in an open culture
- Metal Scale 3 Having purpose and direction
- Meta Scale 3 feeling valued and empowered

Each of these Meta scales is then further made up by two sub-scales, one of which relates to individual aspects of engagement (notation I) and another relating to organisational conditions (notation O).

The prototype Medical Engagement Scale was then piloted with four NHS secondary care trusts. Two of those trusts had been identified and recognised independently for their work on engaging clinicians, another trust was in a state of crisis where a new chief executive suspected that lack of medial engagement was a significant problem and a final volunteer trust was unknown in terms of the likely picture of medical engagement. The Medical Engagement Scale was then given to a sample of all doctors in these trusts (with a 56% return rate overall) as well as a smaller sample of senior managers (non-medical) who were asked to estimate the level of medical engagement they thought existed in their trust.

This resulting data was used to establish a number of key practical and conceptual aspects of the Medical Engagement Scale, notably that:

- the overall and sub-scales were reliable with Cronbach alpha coefficients from .70 to .93
- engagement is part of but distinct from a more general concept of organisational culture
- the new Medical Engagement Scale had face validity, being able to differentiate statistically significant differences between the four pilot trust sites and in precisely the predicted order of engagement, i.e. they were independently identified as outstanding at the top of the engagement scale, with the crisis trust at the bottom and the unknown in between.

Following this relatively successful pilot stage, the Medical Engagement Scale was then applied to a further 30 secondary care trusts in the NHS in order:

- to establish normative data for patterns of medical engagement, and
- to assess the underlying issue relating to medical engagement – does it relate to organisational performance?

An initial set of norms has been established, and these enable the extent and nature of medical engagement within any trust to be benchmarked and compared. Almost 4, 000 doctors are now represented on the database, offering some fascinating insights as to the relative position of different specialties (nationally) or within an organisation and ways of approaching tricky issues such as differences between designated leaders, including medical and clinical directors, as opposed to the wider group of doctors in the trust.

Perhaps even more excitingly, the data enables the key link between the concept of medical engagement (and the index of it) and organisational performance to be examined with sound empirical information. A simple visual way of seeing this relationship is presented in Table 7.1.

TABLE 7.1 Comparison of MES index (30 secondary care trusts) to overall Care Quality Commission (CCQ) ratings

Trust ID (Trust names withheld for confidentiality)	Overall Medical Engagement Scale Index (in descending order)	Overall quality score	Financial management score	CQC - NHS performance ratings 2008/09		
				Core standards score (as a provider of services)	Existing commitment score (as a provider of services)	National priorities score (as a provider of services)
Top 10 Trusts						
21	65.8	Good	Excellent	Fully Met	Fully Met	Good
12	65.2	Good	Good	Fully Met	–	Good
15	63.4	Excellent	Good	Fully Met	Fully Met	Excellent
5	62.0	Excellent	Excellent	Fully Met	Fully Met	Excellent
24	60.8	Good	Excellent	Fully Met	–	Good
1	60.4	Excellent	Excellent	Fully Met	Fully Met	Excellent
10	59.9	Good	Excellent	Almost Met	Fully Met	Good
16	59.8	Good	Fair	Fully Met	Almost Met	Excellent
14	59.7	Excellent	Excellent	Fully Met	Fully Met	Excellent
11	58.8	Excellent	Excellent	Fully Met	Fully Met	Excellent
Bottom 10 Trusts						
25	56.8	Fair	Fair	Almost Met	Fully Met	Poor
4	56.7	Fair	Fair	Almost Met	Fully Met	Fair
22	55.7	Fair	Fair	Partly Met	Almost Met	Good
23	55.3	Fair	Good	Almost Met	Partly Met	Excellent
29	54.4	Good	Excellent	Fully Met	Fully Met	Good
3	54.3	Fair	Excellent	Fully Met	Fully Met	Poor
26	53.1	Fair	Fair	Almost Met	Almost Met	Fair
8	52.7	Good	Good	Fully Met	Almost Met	Good
18	52.1	Fair	Fair	Fully Met	Partly Met	Good
20	47.0	Poor	Poor	Almost Met	Not Met	Fair

Health and Social Care organisations in England are subject to performance monitoring and regulation under the auspices of the Care Quality Commission (CQC) as the regulatory body. The Commission represents an overarching framework bringing together previous NHS Performance Frameworks and the activities of Monitor (the regulator for Foundation Trusts within the overall set of NHS Trusts). The cumulative nature of the development has resulted in a very large number of standards across a range of areas. Performance in each area is rated as Achieved, Underachieved or Failed, and the measure is specific to each particular standard. Some standards are generic and others specific to different types of healthcare providers. Broadly the many standards can be grouped under the following areas:

- Operational standards and Targets, e.g. cancelled operations, meeting waiting targets
- Finance, e.g. utilisation of resources
- User experience, e.g. provision of information, treated with respect
- Quality and safety, e.g. incidents, infection rates.

Ultimately the performance levels are drawn together into overall trust ratings across the main aspects such that trusts are described as weak, fair, good and excellent in their pattern of service provision.

Table 7.1 provides a simple visual exploration of how the top and bottom scoring trusts on the Medical Engagement Index fare on the main CQC ratings (overall quality, financial management, care standards, existing commitments and national priorities). Although slightly less than perfect, it is quite apparent from visual comparison of, for example, overall quality and financial management, that the top 10 medical engagement index trusts are good or excellent, with one exception. In contrast, the bottom 10 medical engagement index trusts are generally fair or poor (weak) with the odd exception in financial management.

Table 7.2 provides specific examples of how particular standards of the CQC correlate with scores on the Medical Engagement Scale, both at the Medical Engagement Index level and also in relation to some of the sub-scales of the measure. Virtually all correlations are significant (and positive) with their level of significance indicated in the Table. Where less than 30 trusts are involved, this is because the particular measure is not applicable to this type of healthcare provider.

A more detailed statistical analysis also reveals a large number of significant relationships between the medical engagement index and other independently collected performance markers. For example, standardised mortality rates correlate significantly at (.01 level) $-.50$ with the overall Engagement Index and $-.50$ with Meta Scale 3 (being valued and empowered) and $-.56$ with Meta Scale 1 (working in a collaborative culture). Similarly, from the National Patient Safety Agency data, overall Medical Engagement ($-.34$) and Meta Scale 2 ($-.46$) correlate significantly with incidents resulting in severe harm.

TABLE 7.2 Care Quality Commission NHS performance ratings

	Medical Engagement Index	Meta 1: Working in a Collaborative Culture	Meta 2: Having Purpose and Direction	Meta 3: Being Valued and Empowered	Sub 1: Climate for Positive Learning	Sub 2: Good Interpersonal Relationships	Sub 3: Appraisal and Rewards Effectively Aligned	Sub 4: Participation in Decision Making and Change	Sub 5: Development Orientation	Sub 6: Work Satisfaction	n Trusts
The Care Quality Commission – NHS performance ratings 2008/09											
Overall quality score	0.68 ***	0.63 ***	0.70 ***	0.65 ***	0.68 ***	0.46 **	0.73 ***	0.49 **	0.62 ***	0.62 ***	30
08/09 financial management score	0.47 **	0.48 **	0.44 **	0.46 **	0.50 **	0.37 *	0.52 **	0.24	0.47 **	0.41 **	30
08/09 core standards score (as a provider of services)	0.34 *	0.37 *	0.25	0.36 *	0.37 *	0.31 *	0.31 *	0.12	0.41 *	0.28	30
08/09 existing commitments score (as a provider of services)	0.64 ***	0.59 ***	0.67 ***	0.60 ***	0.64 ***	0.45 *	0.69 ***	0.53 **	0.61 ***	0.55 **	25

(Continued)

93

TABLE 7.2 Care Quality Commission NHS performance ratings (Continued)

2008/09 NHS performance ratings existing commitments and national priorities indicator scores (frequency of 'achieved')	0.69 ***	0.54 **	0.75 ***	0.70 ***	0.56 **	0.44 *	0.76 ***	0.62 ***	0.66 ***	0.68 ***	25
Total time in A&E: four hours or less (% level 'achievement')	0.55 **	0.55 **	0.47 *	0.59 ***	0.52 **	0.53 **	0.52 **	0.33	0.70 ***	0.46 *	24
Inpatients waiting longer than the 26 week standard (% level 'underachievement')	−0.57 ***	−0.59 ***	−0.41 *	−0.64 ***	−0.52 **	−0.62 ***	−0.44 *	−0.30	−0.72 ***	−0.52 *	25
All cancers: two month urgent referral to treatment (% level 'achievement')	0.54 **	0.52 **	0.42 *	0.61 ***	0.49 **	0.50 **	0.35 *	0.46 *	0.60 ***	0.57 **	24

[1] Attentuated range of performance ratings

Levels of significance; * = p < 0.05, ** = p < 0.01, *** = p < 0.001

This powerful and unique data is evidence of a strong association between levels of medical engagement and externally assessed performance parameters in healthcare providers. This is consistent with much of the earlier literature around engagement reported from other sectors. Although the evidence here is correlational it is difficult to mount the alternative interpretation, i.e. that a disaffected, disillusioned and disengaged medical workforce is likely to lead to sustained high levels of organisational performance. The number, strength and the direction of the correlation is compelling. It is important that the NHS, just as Macleod and Clarke (2009) recommend, recognise the critical role of engagement and seek to identify better ways to nurture and develop it.

LEADING FOR ENGAGEMENT

Returning to the premises of the earlier sections of this chapter, the data on engagement and its link to performance reinforces the crucial role of leaders in creating the appropriate cultures for medical engagement to flourish. Armit and Roberts (2009) recognise this too in detailing the argument that reform and improved performance in health systems is in itself dependent upon fully engaged doctors and that in order for this to happen, the organisational culture, shaped and influenced by its leadership, is going to have to be appropriately supportive and constructive. The acquisition of leadership competence by doctors themselves will form an important element in creating this enhanced engagement.

Building on the evidence of the importance of medical engagement to performance, more recent work has attempted to explore with the top six trusts on the Medical Engagement Scale what they have done to create the engagement and how others may go about enhancing their own existing levels. Although preliminary and based on a limited number of case studies, some consistent themes are emerging.

An interesting structural issue that resonates with the work of Ham (2009), when exploring high-performing organisations internationally, is the stability and hence continuity of the executive team. If engagement is anything, it must be about relationships and it takes time to build trust and respect in a relationship. It is something policymakers might wish to give more consideration. Grand gestures involving the sacking of executives for 'failure' may assuage some kind of public demand for blame and accountability, but on the evidence of the importance of stability in organisations it would seem to be doing little to facilitate sustainable improvement.

More generally, the prescription seems to be that there is a need to build a culture of engagement. As with all cultural change, this may take many forms and be symbolised in the context of a particular situation. However, examples observed in trusts with the highest levels of engagement include:

- **leadership** – stable, top-level leadership that promotes and fosters relationships, sets expectations and leads by example

- **selecting and appointing the right doctors to leadership and management roles** – selecting through open competition ensuring a choice of candidates and appointing based on ability, attitude, leadership aptitude and potential
- **promotion of understanding, trust and respect between doctors and managers** – developing an acknowledgement and acceptance of professional differences, ensuring managers and doctors share a common goal to deliver high quality healthcare to patients
- **clarity of roles and responsibility and empowerment** – ensuring doctors and managers work together, are accountable and empowered to shape and develop the organisation
- **effective communication** – building trust and developing relationships through open, honest communication that is persistent, widespread and inclusive
- **setting expectations, enforcing professional behaviour and firm decision-making** – ensuring organisation expectations are clearly communicated and that issues relating to unprofessional behaviour and patient safety are dealt with quickly and decisively
- **providing support, development and leadership opportunities to doctors at all levels** – investing in training, mentoring and coaching, ensuring formal and informal leadership opportunities are available, spotting and supporting talent, and succession planning
- **developing a future-focussed and outward-looking culture** – encouraging and engaging in best practice, and promoting and contributing at regional and national level.

Each organisation will need to make such initiatives meaningful in their own circumstances, but the crucial role of engagement in supporting organisational achievement suggests the rewards are clear and long-term. The development of such levels of engagement will be crucial to the current coalition government's plans to put clinicians, both primary and secondary, at the forefront of key decision-making in the NHS.

REFERENCES

Alimo-Metcalf B, Bradley M. Cast in a new light. *People Management.* 2008; 24 Jan: 18–23.

Armit K, Roberts H. Engaging doctors: the NHS needs the very best leaders. *Asia Pacific Journal of Health Management.* 2009; 4(2): 47–52.

Atkinson S, Spurgeon P, Clark J, *et al. Engaging Doctors: what can we learn from trusts with high levels of medical engagement.* NHS Institute for Innovation and Improvement and Academy of Royal Colleges: University of Warwick campus, Coventry; 2011.

Bernthal PR. *Measuring Employee Engagement* [White Paper]. Pittsburgh, PA: Development Dimensions International; 2003.

Black C. *Working for a Healthier Tomorrow: review of the health of Britain's working age population.* Available at: www.workingforhealth.gov.uk/documents/working-for-a-healthier-tomorrow-tagged.pdf (accessed 23 April 2011).

Darzi A. *High Quality Care for All: NHS Next Stage Review Final Report.* London: Department of Health; 2008.

Edmonstone J, Western J. Leadership development in healthcare: what do we know? *Journal of Management in Medicine.* 2002; **16**(1): 34–47.

Freeney Y, Tiernan J. Employee engagement: an overview of the literature on the proposed antithesis to burnout. *The Irish Journal of Psychology.* 2006; **27**(3–4): 130–41.

Guthrie M. Engaging physicians in performance improvement. *American Journal of Medical Quality.* 2005; **10**(5) 235–8.

Ham C. Improving the performance of health services: the role of clinical leadership. *Lancet.* 25 March 2003. Available at: http://image.thelancet.com/extras/02art8342web.pdf (accessed 23 April 2011).

Ham C. *Health Policy in Britain.* 6th ed. Basingstoke: Macmillan; 2009b.

Ham C, Dickenson H. *Engaging Doctors in Leadership: review of the literature.* Birmingham: HSMC; 2008.

Harter JK, Schmidt FL, Keyes CLM. Well-being in the workplace and its relationship to business outcomes: a review of the Gallup studies. In: CLM Keyes, J Haidt, editors. *Flourishing: positive psychology and the life well-lived.* Washington DC: American Psychological Association; 205–24.

Harter JK, Schmidt FL, Kilham EA, *et al. Q12 Meta-analysis.* The Gallup Organisation; 2006.

Hauck K, Rice N, Smith P. The influence of healthcare organisations on health system performance. *J Health Services Research Policy.* 2003; **8**(2): 68–74.

Kahn WA. Psychological conditions of personal engagement and disengagement at work. *Academy of Management Journal.* 1990; **33**: 692–724.

Keroack MA, Youngberg BJ, Cerese JL, *et al.* Organisational factors associated with high performance in quality and safety in academic medical centers. *Academic Medicine.* 2007; **82**(12): 1178–86.

Macleod D, Clarke N. Engaging for success: enhancing performance through employee engagement. *Department for Business Innovation & Skills.* Available at: www.bis.gov.uk (accessed 23 April 2011).

Mannion R, Davies H, Marshall M. Impact of star performance ratings in English acute hospital trusts. *J Health Services Research Policy.* 2006; **10**(1): 18–24.

Maslach C, Jackson SE. *Maslach Burnout Inventory.* 2nd ed. Palo Alto, CA: Consulting Psychologists Press; 1986.

Reinertsen JL, Gosfield AG, Rupp W, *et al. Engaging Physicians in a Shared Quality Agenda.* Boston, MA: Innovation Series (IHI); 2007.

Salanova M, Agut J, Piero JM. Linking organisational facilitators and work engagement to employee performance and customer loyalty: the mediation of service climate. *Journal of Applied Psychology.* 2005; **90**: 1217–27.

Schaufeli WB, Bakker AB. *Utrecht Work Engagement Scale: preliminary manual* [version 1]. Utrecht, Netherlands: Occupational Health Psychology Unit, Utrecht University; 2003.

Shipton H, Armstrong C, West M, *et al.* The impact of leadership and quality climate on hospital performance. *Int J Qual Health Care.* 2008; **20**(6): 439–45.

Smith PC. Performance measurement in health care: history, challenges and prospects. *Public Money & Management.* 2005; **25**(4): 213–20.

Sutherland AM, Dodd F. NHS Lanarkshire's leadership development programme's impact on clinical practice. *International Journal of Health Care Quality Assurance.* 2008; **21**(6): 509–84.

Toto DA. *What the Doctor Ordered: the best hospitals create emotional bands with their physicians.* Available at: http://gmj.gallup.com/content/18361/what-doctor-ordered.aspx (accessed 27 May 2011).

Waddell G, Burton AK. *Is Work Good for Your Health and Well-being?* London: The Stationery Office; 2006.

West M, Borrill C, Dawson J, *et al.* The link between the management of employees and patient mortality in acute hospitals. *Int J Hum Resour Man.* 2002; **13**(8): 1299–310.

The development of the Medical Leadership Competency Framework

INTRODUCTION

The purpose of this chapter is to explore the use of competences in medical education, training and practice with a particular focus on the management and leadership competences doctors should attain. Several existing competency frameworks used in practice by the medical and other health professions in both the UK and internationally to inform leadership development are reviewed. It should be noted the review is not comprehensive or representative and is a selective account of apparently relevant models.

COMPETENCES AS THE BASIS FOR MEDICAL TRAINING

Rapid change in the healthcare environment has pressured healthcare organisations and medical professional, regulatory and educational bodies to begin examining more carefully what it means to be a fully competent doctor. As a result, interest in developing and using competences to influence how healthcare professionals are educated, trained and work has increased over the past few decades. Of particular interest is the emphasis on management and leadership competences.

There are various definitions of competency, although all are broadly similar and mainly focused in the workplace situation/job. From a human resources perspective, competency could be defined as the knowledge, skills and attitudes that:

1   affect a major part of one's job (role or responsibility)
2   correlate with performance on the job
3   are measured against well-accepted standards
4   are improved by training and development. (Lucia, Lepsinger, 1999, p. 5)

Wass and van der Vleuten, in Carter and Jackson (2009), define competency in the clinical context as 'the ability to handle a complex professional task by integrating the relevant cognitive, psychomotor and affective skills' (Carter, Jackson, p. 105).

Prior to the introduction and widespread use of competences, intelligence and aptitude tests were commonly used to determine an individual's suitability for particular roles and responsibilities. McClelland (1973) suggested such measurements were unsuitable due to their poor relationship to practical outcomes and proposed that competences would be a more useful approach. Competences have many advantages in that they 'include a broad range of knowledge, attitudes, and observable patterns of behaviour which together account for the ability to deliver a specified professional service' (McGaghie, Miller, Sajid *et al.*, 1978, p. 19) and can be used to apply to a range of professions and career levels or stages. These are often called core competences and are described as being associated with the success of the organisation as they are more general, flexible and can be adapted according to changing organisational needs and strategy (Garman, Johnson, 2006).

The adoption of competences in the workplace has resulted in their use as forming the basis of curricula and assessment in education and training of professionals. The other driver has been an increasing demand from those who provide the funds for medical education and those who depend on the services delivered by its graduates to make the educational process more in line with health needs of the population (McGaghie, Miller, Sajid *et al.*, 1978).

In 1978 the World Health Organization published a paper entitled *Competency-Based Curriculum Development in Medical Education* (McGaghie, Miller, Sajid *et al.*), which described the evolution of medical curriculum from being centred on individual clinical disciplines or subjects, through to a more integrated model, and eventually to being competency-based. They explained that the 'intended output of a competency-based curriculum is a health professional who can practise medicine at a defined level of proficiency in accord with local conditions to meet local needs' (McGaghie, Miller, Sajid *et al.*, 1978, p. 20). The authors also highlighted that the key differences of a competency-based curriculum compared to a subject-based or integrated curriculum are that it is:

1 'organised around functions (or competences) required for the practice of medicine in a specified setting
2 grounded in the empirically validated principle that students of the intellectual quality found in medical schools, when given appropriate instruction, can all master the prescribed basic performance objectives
3 based on a view of education as an experiment where both the process of student learning and the techniques used to produce learning are regarded as hypothesis subject to testing' (McGaghie, Miller, Sajid *et al.*, 1978, p. 18).

In addition, the authors cite numerous benefits of a competency-based curriculum, including:

- a more comprehensive curriculum that can deal with issues such as 'administrative leadership, liaison with governmental bodies, social research and consumer education' (p. 22)
- a competent doctor that uses the knowledge of physical and biological sciences and comprehension of social and cultural factors that influence patient care and well-being to perform clinical tasks (p. 19)

- opportunity for cumulative learning as experience grows along with flexible formative assessment throughout training (p. 19), e.g. in the form of portfolios. This demonstrates that assessing competency is a process of measuring integrated, not isolated, skills. (In the UK, the former Postgraduate Medical Education and Training Board (PMETB)[1] required medical royal colleges to review specialty curricula and assessment to ensure concentration on supportive, formative and reflective systems)
- Clear end-points of summative assessment demonstrating that competence has been achieved. (p. 19)

In 2002, the first competency-based curriculums were published by the three Royal Colleges of Physicians in the UK (Joint Committee for Higher Medical Training). These represented a restructuring of training and assessment for specialist registrars. The curricula were based on achieving a range of competences considered necessary for doctors to work as independent consultants. Knowledge, skills and attitudes required for each competency were described. Assessment for each competency was also defined and was to be continuous, on the job, with tutors cross-checking knowledge and experience (Mayor, 2002).

The process of acquiring or developing competence or defining the different levels of competence development can be described using Miller's pyramid (Miller, 1990) (Figure 8.1) or Bloom's taxonomy (Bloom, 1956) (Table 8.1).

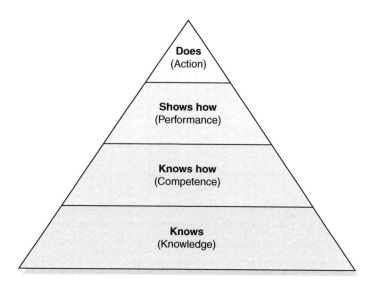

FIGURE 8.1 Miller's pyramid

---

[1] PMETB was the independent regulatory body responsible for postgraduate medical education and training until its assimilation into the GMC in 2010. It aims to ensure that postgraduate training for doctors is of the highest standard.

TABLE 8.1 Bloom's taxonomy

Level	Description
1	Knowledge – specifics, ways and means to deal, universal or abstract principles in a field
2	Comprehension – grasping meaning
3	Application – using information in concrete/specific situations
4	Analysis – ability to break material into its parts
5	Synthesis – putting part together into a whole
6	Evaluation – judging the value of something for a given purpose using predefined criteria

For Miller's pyramid, from the base of the pyramid upwards, *knows* indicates basic knowledge, *knows how* is applied knowledge (highlighting that there is more to clinical competence than knowledge alone), *shows how* represents a behavioural function, and *does* tests performance. This system is often used in assessment of skills and performance in medicine.

Bloom's taxonomy, however, focuses more on cognitive knowledge than performance.

In developing core competences which apply to healthcare professionals, Shewcuk, O'Connor and Fine (2005) highlight several important factors worthy of consideration. Firstly, there are often numerous organisational settings in terms of focus and mission; for example, doctors can work in many different settings from primary care to acute, mental health, third sector, etc.

Secondly, in healthcare there are multiple professions with their own knowledge and skills based on numerous disciplines and specialties. For doctors in the UK, there is a choice of 57 different specialties! That said, in many cases more than one profession and more than one specialty will have or use some of the same body of knowledge in a particular field.

Thirdly, different competences may emerge at different points along a career trajectory. For a medical student, opportunities to develop and demonstrate particular competences will be different to those of a doctor in training or a consultant or GP; therefore they will develop over time through their education, training and practice.

Fourthly, healthcare is a context-specific field. If competences are removed from specific contexts and actual behaviours have almost no meaning in terms of how they relate to important outcomes and objectives of training, they are unlikely to have value. Furthermore, Shewcuk *et al.* (2005) contend that competences not embedded in a framework are likely to be of little lasting value.

McGaghie *et al.* (1978) make an important point that the 'definition of medical competence is bound to local political, social, and economic circumstances, to health needs, to the availability of resources, and to the structure of the health care system' (p. 23). In the UK, the Academy of Medical Royal Colleges and NHS

Institute for Innovation and Improvement have worked in conjunction with the medical professional bodies and health service to define the management and leadership competences required of doctors in their practitioner roles.

COMPETENCY FRAMEWORKS IN THE UK

There have been a number of reviews and publications from within the medical profession, e.g. the British Medical Association, 2004; General Medical Council, 2006; Royal College of Surgeons, 2007, which focus on non-clinical competences,[2] the managerial role of doctors, and the effective management of doctors by doctors (Davies, Hodges, Rundall *et al.*, 2003).

In addition, there have been multiple studies that have developed generic competency frameworks for all levels of doctors in training, those at the consultant level and for senior clinical manager-leader roles, i.e. clinical and medical directors and professional executive committee (PEC) chairs. The essential message from these studies is that sufficient clinical knowledge and skill is the baseline; however, for a doctor to be an effective and safe practitioner in a complex health system requires an additional range of non-clinical competences, including management and leadership.

In the UK, management and leadership has not generally been considered part of the core undergraduate curriculum (medical school) as the focus is on the clinical skills necessary to become a competent doctor. However, many elements of what could be considered management and leadership, e.g. communication, teamwork, and self-awareness, have historically been taught under different headings such as professionalism or personal and professional development. Some student-selected modules introduce the concepts of leadership and management outside the core curriculum. However, until recently, there has been a lack of a comprehensive and common framework for these competences.

At foundation stage, most training has been through in-house arrangements with postgraduate deaneries and NHS trusts.. The curriculum for the foundation programme (www.foundationprogramme.nhs.uk/pages/home/key-documents#curriculum) details a series of core professional competences that cover 14 areas:

1 professionalism
2 good clinical care
3 recognition and management of the acutely ill patient
4 resuscitation
5 discharge and planning for chronic disease management
6 relationship with patients and communications skills
7 patient safety within clinical governance
8 infection control
9 nutritional care

---

[2]The terms 'non-clinical competences', 'non-medical competences', 'management competences' and 'leadership competences' seem to be used interchangeably to some extent, but all cover similar areas related to a range of applied skills and knowledge necessary to be effective in the complex organisational systems required to deliver healthcare.

10 health promotion, patient education and public health
11 ethical and legal issues
12 maintaining good medical practice
13 teaching and training
14 working with colleagues.

Leadership is explicitly mentioned under 'professionalism' and 'working with colleagues'.

During the postgraduate or specialty training stage, the emphasis has historically been on developing doctors for the future. While there are some specific programmes on management and leadership offered by deaneries locally, many doctors did not access these programmes until the final six months of their specialty training in preparation for appointment to a GP or consultant post.

Currently, development and assessment of generic skills has not been robust or consistent enough throughout this stage, and there is general agreement by medical leadership and health policymakers that all doctors, regardless of specialty, should have a minimum set of management and leadership skills to be able to fulfil their practitioner roles more effectively.

Once a doctor is appointed to a consultant or GP position in the UK they ipso facto become leaders within the health system – not necessarily in formal leadership roles but as professionals who are expected to give a lead both by the health and wider community. Over the past decade, there has been a much clearer understanding and acceptance of the need for qualified doctors to have developed, or to rapidly acquire, a range of leadership and managerial competences.

In the UK, until 2008, there has been no one common and recognised management and leadership competency framework for doctors, although a number of papers and frameworks have been published in recent years by a variety of medical and non-medical organisations.

The General Medical Council (GMC)[3] published *Management for Doctors* in February 2006, and it sets out the competences and standards that define a good medical manager. At the time of writing, the GMC were consulting on updated guidance, *Good Management Practice: guidance for all doctors*.

Medical professional organisations have also published guidelines on management and leadership for doctors. The British Medical Association (BMA)[4] in *Developing the Doctor-Manager Leadership Role* (2004) uses Allen's (1995) descriptions of four levels of medical management, with each level requiring a different complement of skills and leadership becoming an increasingly key component through the levels.

---

[3]The General Medical Council (GMC) registers doctors to practise medicine in the UK. The purpose is to protect, promote and maintain the health and safety of the public by ensuring proper standards in the practice of medicine. www.gmc-uk.org

[4]The British Medical Association is the independent trade union and professional association for doctors and medical students, with over 140 000 members in the United Kingdom and overseas. www.bma.org.uk

The Management Standards Centre (MSC)[5] is the UK government-recognised standards-setting body for management and leadership areas. The MSC developed a new set of *National Occupational Standards (NOS) for Management and Leadership* in 2008, which describe the level of performance expected in employment for a range of management and leadership functions/activities. The standards are designed to provide a framework for the development of qualifications and to support a wide range of human resource management and development purposes including aiding decisions on recruitment, selection and recognition and development of future leaders (*see* www.management-standards.org.uk). The NOS can be used for all health professionals; however, unlike the Leadership Qualities Framework (LQF) below, there is no specific application for doctors.

There are broad similarities in the competences, standards or qualities identified in each of the above frameworks around personal qualities, interactions with others and working within and across the organisation. Several of the documents identified the need to focus on personal qualities in terms of self-belief, management, awareness, development and integrity. Interactions with people varied from statements around just working with others to recruiting; leading; managing and developing staff, colleagues, trainees, etc. by empowering and developing their skills. Department and organisational statements focused on delivering and improving services; driving for outcomes and achieving results; managing and developing the business through planning use of and managing resources, e.g. financial; identifying and setting objectives; managing projects and managing change. Furthermore, some frameworks highlighted the importance of decision-making and providing direction either at local or strategic level and therefore the need to understand the wider context. Other statements were around communication, patient safety, equality, diversity, opportunity and quality.

Even if not explicitly stated, most frameworks, e.g. *A Syllabus for Doctors in Leadership and Management Positions in Healthcare* (2007), have been intended for individuals, including doctors, who are already in formal leadership roles and aiming for executive-level positions. These were probably the most comprehensive and developed competency frameworks until the development of the Medical Leadership Competency Framework (discussed in the following section), which is intended for all doctors as part of their practitioner roles.

COMPETENCY FRAMEWORKS IN OTHER COUNTRIES

Other countries with similar histories of low medical engagement in planning, delivery and transformation of services are also recognising that improvements to

---

[5]The Management Standards Centre aims to fulfil the needs of employers by developing a skilled management workforce through promoting our nationally recognised set of standards and qualifications, which have full employer relevance and 'ownership'. www.management-standards.org.uk

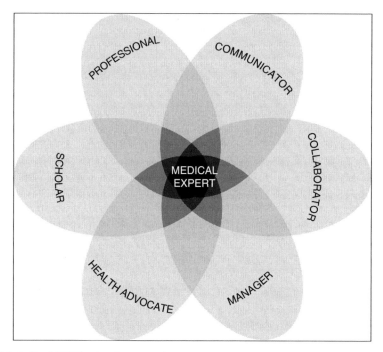

FIGURE 8.2 CanMEDS roles framework

the health system are unlikely to be realised without creating organisational cultures that encourage doctors to want to be involved. This requires a paradigm shift in how the medical profession sees the future role of the doctor and thus how they are trained in the future. Both Denmark and Canada stand out in their approach to defining the role of a doctor and the competences required, including management and leadership, to be effective practitioners.

As noted briefly in Chapter 6, the Royal College of Physicians and Surgeons of Canada[6] developed the CanMEDS Roles Framework and associated competences (Figure 8.2). CanMEDS 'is a competency framework, a guide to the essential abilities physicians need for optimal patient outcomes' (Frank, 2005, p. 1). It 'forms the basis of the standards of the educational mission of the royal college and has been incorporated into accreditation, evaluation and examinations, as well as objectives of training and standards for continuing professional development' (Frank, 2005, p. 1). It can be used by educators, teachers, trainees, practising physicians, researchers and other healthcare professionals. Importantly, it can be used as the 'basis for medical curricula and throughout the physician's learning continuum, beginning at undergraduate level, during residency and continuing professional development' (Frank, 2005, p. v).

[6]The Royal College of Physicians and Surgeons of Canada is a national organization responsible for setting and maintaining the standards for postgraduate medical education, for certifying specialist physicians and surgeons in Canada, and for promoting their continuing education. www.royalcollege.ca

These are six roles with associated competences that combine to provide a central role of 'medical expert'. These are outlined in the model in Figure 8.2.

CanMEDS is not a medical management and leadership group of competences. It is set at a high level of description, and implies a range of underlying sub-sets of competences in terms of how these would actually be achieved in practice through the application of specific skills and knowledge to particular situations. However, two of the role-related competency sets, the collaborator and the manager, have a more managerial aspect.

The Board of the National Union of Consultants in the Danish Medical Association[7] has also developed a model of leadership, which include five leadership core competences:

- personal leadership
- leadership in a political context
- leading quality
- leading change
- leading professionals.

They also include eight roles for the consultant as a professional leader (these are similar to the CanMEDs roles):

- medical expert
- professional
- leader/administrator
- academic
- collaborator
- communicator
- promoter of health
- adviser
  (The Danish Medical Association, 2006).

These roles are part of the Danish medical culture and influence behaviours and curriculum, and also form appointment criteria. The curricula at both undergraduate and postgraduate levels are based around these eight roles. This includes mandatory training in management and leadership before the equivalent of a Certificate of Completion of Training (CCT)[8] is awarded, providing access to apply for consultant and general practitioner positions. Immediately after appointment, all new hospi-

---

[7]The specific objectives of the DMA, as stated in its statutes, are: to unite Danish doctors in order to protect the interests of the medical profession, and to serve as the body through which the influence of the medical profession may be exercised on general social issues in the best interest of health and the healthcare system. www.laeger.dk

[8]CCT or Certificate of Completion of Training is the certificate that physicians in the United Kingdom receive to indicate that they have completed training in their chosen specialty and are eligible to apply for a post as a consultant or a general practitioner (GP). http://en.wikipedia.org/wiki/Certificate_of_Completion_of_Training

tal consultants are expected, as part of their continuous professional development, to participate in further leadership development programmes jointly run by the Association of County Councils in Denmark and the Danish Medical Association, e.g. 'You are a good clinician – are you a good leader too?'.

Research has also been undertaken in Australia and the United States into the key competences doctors should have in their management and leadership roles. The Royal Australasian College of Medical Administrators (RACMA)[9] identified communication, personal leadership skills, ability to engage medical staff, strategic thinking and analytical skills to be important competences for medical managers to have. This reflected a heightening of significance of these competences along with emphasis on quality and safety nationally and internationally, and has resulted in an increased focus on clinical governance activities such as risk management, quality and performance management for medical leaders. Additionally, new medical-management structures in large health organisations have put more emphasis on strategic health service issues and funding for medical leaders.

There appears to be a diversity of models and approaches to medical leadership and management in the United States, which may be a reflection of the variety of organisations and systems of provision. However, 'competency or outcome based education has been increasingly examined and endorsed by many educational accreditation and professional certification bodies across the health professions' (Calhoun *et al.*, 2008, p. 376). A study in 2004 of the development of physician leadership competences, conducted by McKenna, Gartland and Pugno, identified nine competences of high importance for physician leaders. In rank order these were:

- 'interpersonal and communication skills
- professional ethics and social responsibility
- continuous learning and improvement
- ability to build coalitions and support for change
- clinical excellence
- ability to convey a clear compelling vision
- system based decision making/problem solving
- ability to address needs of multiple stakeholders
- financial acumen and resource management' (p. 348).

In terms of how competence is developed, Mayo Clinic[10] found, through a needs survey of managing and consulting staff physicians and external survey of other organisations and programmes, that a combination of traditional academic

---

[9]RACMA is the body responsible for setting educational standards, training and examination of medical administrators in Australia and New Zealand, leading to the award of Fellowship – FRACMA – a recognised specialist qualification for the medically qualified manager.

[10]Mayo Clinic is the world's oldest and largest multispecialty group practice. It is a world-renowned specialist centre of excellence that has expanded from its base in Minnesota to provide care in Arizona and Florida. Mayo's focus is on patient care, research and education. www.mayoclinic.org

approaches and contextually embedded, personally relevant, behaviourally based experiential learning is essential for the successful development of physician leadership competences (Tangalos, Bloomberg, Bender, 1998).

Competency frameworks have also been developed in Canada and the US that are applicable to all professions, including doctors. The HealthCare Leaders' Association of British Columbia (HCLABC)[11] developed a *Health Leadership Capabilities Framework for Senior Executive Leaders* (2007) and the National Centre for Healthcare Leadership (NCHL)[12] in the United States developed a *Health Leadership Competency Model* (HLCM). Both frameworks aim to define the behaviours, key skills, abilities and knowledge/technical competences of capable leaders. They can also be used to inform education and professional development. Importantly, the *Health Leadership Capabilities Framework for Senior Executive Leaders* (2007) explicitly states that it is based on distributed leadership where everyone, regardless of role or formal position, 'must be able to lead themselves, engage others, achieve results, develop coalitions, and conduct systems transformation' (HealthCare Leaders' Association of British Columbia, p. 3).

All the frameworks and research mentioned broadly focus on competence that contributes to leadership ability and success in healthcare at the individual level, e.g. communication; management skills; engaging, working with and leading others; being a role model and analysing and strategic thinking. Those that are particularly aimed at doctors also recognise the professional role of the doctor as medical expert or in terms of clinical excellence.

Until recently, there was clearly no one framework that addressed the undergraduate, postgraduate and continuing practice management and leadership areas of a doctor's practitioner role either in the UK or internationally. The Medical Leadership Competency Framework (MLCF) developed by the Academy of Medical Royal Colleges, and the NHS Institute is the first management and leadership competency framework that the writers know to be applicable to all stages of a doctor's training and career. Several of the frameworks mentioned above were influential in the development of the MLCF.

THE MEDICAL LEADERSHIP COMPETENCY FRAMEWORK (MLCF)

The MLCF was first published in 2008 and has subsequently been refined. The MLCF describes 'the leadership competences doctors need to become more actively

[11]The HealthCare Leaders' Association of BC is a professional association of leaders in British Columbia's healthcare system and related organizations. www.hclabc.bc.ca
[12]The National Center for Healthcare Leadership (NCHL) is a not-for-profit organization that works to assure that high-quality, relevant and accountable leadership is available to meet the challenges of delivering quality patient healthcare in the 21st century. NCHL's goal is to improve health system performance and the health status of the entire country through effective healthcare management leadership. www.nchl.org/ns/index.asp

involved in the planning, delivery and transformation of health services as a normal part of their role as doctors'. (NHS Institute for Innovation and Improvement, Academy of Medical Royal Colleges, 2010, p. 6).

The purpose of the MLCF was to provide the medical profession, health service and individual doctors with the key management and leadership competences expected of doctors. Although some of these competences may have been previously implicit in medical education and training, the MLCF aims to make them explicit and reduce the variability between medical schools and specialties in how much emphasis these are given.

It was proposed that the MLCF could help inform the design of education and training curricula and development programmes, enable doctors to identify individual strengths and development areas through self-assessment and structured feedback from colleagues and assist with personal development planning and career progression.

The document was designed to complement and build on a range of existing standards and frameworks published by the Department of Health and key medical organisations such as the GMC.

A significant aspect of the MLCF is that it is based on the concept of shared leadership 'where leadership is not restricted to people who hold designated leadership roles, and where there is a shared sense of responsibility for the success of the organisation and its services' (NHS Institute for Innovation and Improvement, Academy of Medical Royal Colleges, 2010, p. 6) and as described in Chapter 3.

How the MLCF was developed is also an important contributor to the wide acceptance and use it has gained in the UK and interest received internationally. The highly inclusive nature by which it was developed involved extensive consultation with key members of the medical and wider NHS community through interviews, reference groups, focus groups, patient groups and a steering group of the top leaders from a wide range of medical bodies. It was also informed by a literature review, comparative analysis of existing leadership competency frameworks and specialty curricula (the latter to identify current provision and any variations or gaps) and review of key medical professional documents. In addition, the developing framework was tested in a variety of medical and service communities. These processes have ensured the leadership competences were positioned within the reality of working in healthcare in the UK today. It also ensured that the language used is appropriate and meaningful to the medical profession.

Delivering services to patients, service users, carers and the public is at the heart of the MLCF. There are five domains of the MLCF (Figure 8.3), and it is considered essential that every doctor is competent in each domain to deliver appropriate, safe and effective services. Within each domain there are four elements (Table 8.2), and each of these is further divided into four competency outcomes.

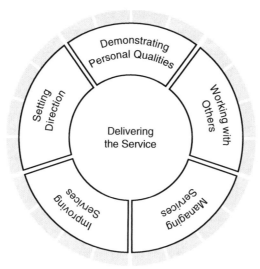

FIGURE 8.3 Medical Leadership Competency Framework (NHS Institute for Innovation and Improvement, Academy of Medical Royal Colleges, 2010, p. 6)

The competences in the MLCF are supported by examples and scenarios that demonstrate how competence can be developed through everyday training and clinical practice at each stage of a doctor's career – undergraduate education, postgraduate training and within the first five years of a doctor becoming a consultant or GP (continuing practice). The MLCF emphasises that the way a doctor demonstrates competence and ability will vary according to the career path chosen and their level of experience and training. An important distinction with other existing frameworks discussed in the previous section is that the MLCF applies to all medical students and doctors as practitioners.

At *undergraduate* stage (medical school) all medical students will be expected to attain learning outcomes as defined by the medical school curriculum (based on the GMC's *Tomorrow's Doctors*). During their medical school training, students will have access to relevant learning opportunities within a variety of situations, e.g. during peer interaction, group learning or clinical placements, which can provide opportunities to develop leadership experience, to develop their personal styles and abilities, and to understand how effective leadership will have an impact on the system and benefit patients as students move from learner to practitioner on graduating (NHS Institute for Innovation and Improvement, Academy of Medical Royal Colleges, 2010, p. 8).

At *postgraduate* stage the MLCF applies to all doctors in training and practice, that is during foundation years and for those in specialty training – where specialty curriculum was approved by the former Postgraduate Medical Education and Training Board (PMETB) – and in non-specialist training posts, i.e. staff grade and associate specialist doctors (under the responsibility of the postgraduate deanery and health

TABLE 8.2 MLCF domains and elements (NHS Institute for Innovation and Improvement, Academy of Medical Royal Colleges, 2010, p. 11)

Domain	Elements
Demonstrating personal qualities	• Developing self-awareness • Managing yourself • Continuing personal development • Acting with integrity
Working with others	• Developing networks • Building and maintaining relationships • Encouraging contribution • Working within teams
Managing services	• Planning • Managing resources • Managing people • Managing performance
Improving services	• Ensuring patient safety • Critically evaluating • Encouraging improvement and innovation • Facilitating transformation
Setting direction	• Identifying the contexts for change • Applying knowledge and evidence • Making decisions • Evaluating impact

service). (NHS Institute for Innovation and Improvement, Academy of Medical Royal Colleges, 2010, p. 8).

As doctors train and consolidate their skills and knowledge in everyday practice, they are very often the key medical person relating with other staff and experiencing how day-to-day healthcare works in action. They are therefore uniquely placed to develop experience in management and leadership through relationships with other people, departments and ways of working, and to understand how the patient experiences healthcare, and how the processes and systems of delivering care can be improved. Specific activities such as clinical audit and research also offer the opportunity to learn management and leadership skills. With all this comes the need to understand how their specialty and focus of care contributes to the wider healthcare system (NHS Institute for Innovation and Improvement, Academy of Medical Royal Colleges, 2010, p. 8).

Continuing practice describes the stage of post-specialist certification, or the time during the first years of practice after training. The MLCF applies to all consultants and general practitioners. It also applies to doctors who do not have specialist or generalist registration but who work as staff or associate specialist grade or as trust doctors in non-career grade posts in hospitals (NHS Institute for Innovation and Improvement, Academy of Medical Royal Colleges, 2010, p. 9).

The end of the formal training period brings with it roles and responsibilities within the team delivering patient care, as well as in the wider healthcare system. Doctors require an understanding of the need for each area to play its part. Experienced doctors develop their abilities in leadership within their departments and practices and by working with colleagues in other settings and on projects. Familiarity with their specific focus of care enables them to work outside their immediate setting and to look further at ways to improve the experience of healthcare for patients and colleagues. As established members of staff or partners, they are able to develop further their leadership abilities by actively contributing to the running of the organisation and to the way care is generally provided (NHS Institute for Innovation and Improvement, Academy of Medical Royal Colleges, 2010, p. 9).

The following graphics show the emphasis that is likely to be given to the MLCF domains at each stage of career progression.

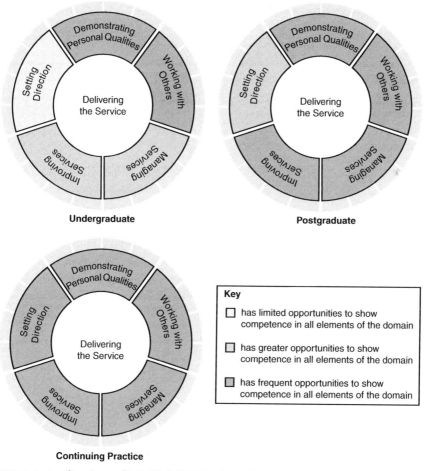

FIGURE 8.4 Application of MLCF (NHS Institute for Innovation and Improvement, Academy of Medical Royal Colleges, 2010, p. 8–9)

By the end of the undergraduate stage, it is expected that competence should have been developed in all aspects of Demonstrating Personal Qualities and Working with Others. There will have been less opportunity for undergraduates to demonstrate competence in all aspects of the other three domains, particularly Setting Direction. However, they should at least have developed the underpinning knowledge and skills as a foundation for future competence in these areas (NHS Institute for Innovation and Improvement, Academy of Medical Royal Colleges, 2010, p. 8–9).

Integrating the MLCF into curricula at undergraduate and postgraduate levels will ensure medical students and doctors are developing competence in management and leadership early in their career and make it compulsory, rather than an optional extra. The implication of this is that a medical student or doctor will not be able to progress to the next career stage without demonstrating competence in management and leadership.

As mentioned previously, the GMC document *Tomorrow's Doctors* now incorporates all competences of the MLCF, albeit in slightly different language, and makes the requirement of developing management and leadership skills more explicit for undergraduates. This requires all medical schools in the UK to demonstrate that the competences are included and assessed in their undergraduate curricula.

The competences have also been incorporated into each Medical Royal College's specialty curriculum. The specialty curriculum outlines the competences trainees need to attain in order to secure a Certificate of Completion of Training. As the regulatory body responsible at the time for approving curricula, PMETB stated that they would expect to see the MLCF competences and appropriate assessment methods, e.g. multisource feedback and case-based discussion, integrated into specialty curricula.

One of the implications of integration into curricula is that those responsible for medical education and training will be required to deliver the management and leadership element of the curriculum and assess management and leadership competence in medical students and doctors in training. The ability and competence of clinical tutors and medical educationalists is crucial to ensuring doctors learn management and leadership in the context of their everyday clinical practice. Furthermore, doctors learn from other doctors and the importance of role models should not be underestimated.

As the MLCF competences are embedded in undergraduate and postgraduate curricula there will be a stronger expectation over the coming years that when doctors apply for consultant or general practitioner posts they will be able to demonstrate competence in management and leadership. Indeed, there is an expectation now that doctors can demonstrate such competence. However, organisations are likely to consider this a key part of recruitment decisions in the future, particularly as organisations know that they are recruiting a consultant or general practitioner for many years and want to ensure they are getting the right person, with the right skills and drive to develop and improve services for patients and enhance organisational performance.

Management and leadership competences are also likely to be given more emphasis during annual appraisal so doctors continue to demonstrate how their management and leadership skills are contributing to patient services, the organisation and system within which they work.

The UK medical profession is currently introducing revalidation, whereby doctors will need to demonstrate on a regular basis that they practice in accordance with GMC's generic standards and they meet the standards appropriate to their specialty (*see* www.gmc-uk.org/doctors/revalidation.asp). As the competences are integrated into specialty curriculum and into the GMC's core guidance for doctors, *Good Medical Practice*, it is likely that competence in management and leadership will need to be demonstrated as part of revalidation.

Healthcare organisations may also explore more joint management and leadership development opportunities for doctors and managers. This will help facilitate the process of cultural change, and may also be of benefit to other clinical professions. Indeed, the successful introduction and application of competency-based leadership and management education and training in the UK may provide a useful model for other countries to adopt elsewhere. This is explored further in Chapter 9.

The implementation of the MLCF in education, training and practice will help support the development of learning opportunities that are timely and relevant to all medical students and doctors. In accepting that the acquisition of leadership and management skills are core for all doctors, the MLCF affords the possibility to deliver appropriate learning outcomes within core clinical training, rather than as a peripheral or extracurricular activity.

CONCLUSION

Clearly many organisations in the UK and elsewhere have gone to great effort to develop their own leadership framework despite a degree of similarity with others that already existed. This probably indicates that the process by which a framework is developed, and the resulting buy-in and ownership from key players that comes from a highly inclusive approach, is what is important.

Improving the health of the population, and the delivery and effectiveness of health and social care services, depends heavily on the support and active engagement of all doctors, not only in their practitioner activities but also in their managerial and leadership roles.

Embedding management and leadership competences in curricula and learning pathways will enable all clinicians to actively contribute to the planning, delivery and transformation of health services for patients.

As the development of management and leadership competence becomes an integral part of doctors' training and learning, all doctors will have a minimum set of management and leadership competence in the future, thereby enhancing their effectiveness. Although not all doctors will want to move into formal leadership positions (for example, clinical director or medical director) it will provide a basic leadership toolkit to enable all doctors to develop further if they wish. On the other hand, it may stimulate more doctors to take on service improvement and executive leadership roles. Hopefully it will also encourage more non-clinical leaders to recognise the importance of real engagement and to be involved in creating cultures and incentives that value the contribution of all doctors.

It is important to recognise that attainment of leadership competence will span across 15+ years of doctors' training, and that leadership competences developed for doctors are now likely to be applied to other clinical professionals.

The integration and application of the MLCF into undergraduate and postgraduate curricula, health service organisations and revalidation will require further development of appropriate assessment methodologies, and an ongoing commitment by the medical education community and regulatory bodies to pursue a competency based approach to examination and accreditation of leadership skills for all doctors. It will also have a long-term and significant impact on the way in which doctors are trained and recruited in the 21st century. To be deemed an effective and safe doctor, all doctors in the UK will be required to attain competence in clinical as well as management and leadership skills.

REFERENCES

Allen D. Doctors in management or the revenge of the conquered – the role of management development for doctors. *Journal of Management in Medicine.* 1995; 9(4): 44–50.

BAMM. *A Syllabus for Doctors in Leadership and Management Positions in Healthcare.* Cheadle: The British Association of Medical Managers; 2007.

Bloom BS. *Taxonomy of Educational Objectives.* New York, NY: Longman; 1956.

British Medical Association. Developing the doctor-manager leadership role. 2004. Available at: www.bma.org.uk/images/Drmanager_tcm41-20460.pdf (accessed 1 April 2009).

Calhoun JG, Dollet L, Sinioris ME, *et al.* Development of Interprofessional Competency Model for Healthcare Leadership. *Journal of Healthcare Management.* 2008; 53(6): 375–90.

Davies HT, Hodges CL, Rundall TG, *et al.* Views of doctors and managers on the doctor-manager relationship in the NHS. *BMJ.* 2003; 326(7390): 626–8.

Frank JR, editor. *The CanMEDS Physician Competency Framework. Better standards. Better physicians. Better care.* Ottawa, ON: The Royal College of Physicians and Surgeons of Canada; 2005.

Garman AN, Johnson MP. Leadership competencies: an introduction. *Journal of Healthcare Management.* 2006; 51(1): 13–18.

General Medical Council. *Good Medical Practice.* Manchester: General Medical Council; 2006a. Available at: www.gmc-uk.org/guidance/good_medical_practice.asp (accessed 1 April 2009).

General Medical Council. *Management for Doctors.* Manchester: General Medical Council; 2006b. Available at: www.gmc-uk.org/guidance/current/library/management_for_doctors.asp (accessed 1 April 2009).

General Medical Council. *Revalidation.* Manchester: General Medical Council; 2006c. Available at: www.gmc-uk.org/doctors/revalidation.asp (accessed 1 April 2009).

General Medical Council. *Tomorrow's Doctors: recommendations on undergraduate medical education.* Manchester: General Medical Council; 2009. Available at: www.gmc-uk.org/education/undergraduate/tomorrows_doctors_2009.asp (accessed 14 April 2010).

Health Care Leaders' Association of British Columbia. *Health Leadership Capabilities Framework.* Victoria, BC: Health Care Leaders' Association of British Columbia; 2007.

Health Care Leaders' Association of British Columbia. *Leaders for Life: Health Leadership Capabilities Framework for senior executive leaders.* Victoria, BC: Health Care Leaders Association of British Columbia; 2007.

Lucia AD, Lepsinger R. *The Art and Science of Competency Models: pinpointing critical success factors in organisations.* San Francisco, CA: Jossey-Bass/Pfeiffer; 1999.

Management Standards Centre. *National Occupational Standards for Management and Leadership.* London: Management Standards Centre; 2008.

Mayor S. UK royal colleges publish competency based curriculums. *BMJ.* 2002; **325**(7377): 1378.

McClelland DC. Testing for competence rather than 'intelligence'. *American Psychologists.* 1973; **28**(1): 1–14.

McGaghie WC, Miller GE, Sajid AW, *et al. Competency-Based Curriculum Development in Medical Education: an introduction* [Public Health Papers No. 68]. Geneva: World Health Organization; 1978.

McKenna M, Gartland P, Pugno P. Development of physician leadership competencies: perceptions of physician leaders, physician educators and medical students. *J Health Adm Educ.* 2004; **21**(3): 343–54.

Miller GE. The assessment of clinical skills/competence/performance. *Acad Med.* 1990; **65**(9): s63–7.

National Centre for Healthcare Leadership. *Health Leadership Competency Model.* Chicago, IL: National Centre for Healthcare Leadership; 2010.

NHS Institute for Innovation and Improvement, Academy of Medical Royal Colleges. *Medical Leadership Competency Framework.* 3rd ed. Coventry: NHS Institute for Innovation and Improvement; 2010.

Postgraduate Medical Education and Training Board (PMETB). *Generic Standards for Training.* London: PMETB; 2008.

Shewcuk RM, O'Connor SJ, Fine DJ. Building an understanding of the competencies needed for health administration practice. *J Healthc Manag.* 2005 Jan-Feb; **50**: 32–49. Available at: www.entrepreneur.com/tradejournals/article/128166399.html (accessed 14 April 2010).

Tangalos EG, Bloomberg RA, Hicks SS, *et al.* Mayo leadership programs for physicians. *Mayo Clin Proc.* 1998 Mar; **73**(3): 279–84.

The Danish Medical Association. *Education for Physician Leadership and Management in Denmark – OLAU.* Copenhagen: The Danish Medical Association; 2006.

The Royal Australasian College of Medical Administrators (RACMA). *RACMA Workforce Report: factors affecting recruitment and retention of medical managers in Australian hospitals*. Malvern: RACMA; 2006.

The Royal College of Physicians and Surgeons of Canada. *The CanMEDS Project Overview*. Ottawa, ON: The Royal College of Physicians and Surgeons of Canada; 2005a.

The Royal College of Physicians and Surgeons of Canada. *CanMEDS 2005 Framework – Key Competences* [draft 5]. Ottawa, ON: The Royal College of Physicians and Surgeons of Canada; 2005b.

The Royal College of Surgeons of England. *The Leadership and Management of Surgical Team*. England: The Royal College of Surgeons of England; 2007.

Wass V, van der Vleuten C. Assessment in medical education and training. In: Carter Y, Jackson N, editors. *Medical Education and Training: From theory to delivery*. Oxford: Oxford University Press; 2009.

CHAPTER 9

Practical examples of initiatives to embed leadership development

Earlier chapters have outlined the various professional, policy and political drivers to secure greater medical engagement in management, leadership and transformation of services. Chapter 8 described the development of the Medical Leadership Competency Framework (MLCF) (NHS Institute for Innovation and Improvement, Academy of Medical Royal Colleges, 2010) and how it is being embedded into undergraduate and postgraduate curricula and being incorporated into revalidation standards for consultants and general practitioners.

In this chapter we explore some of the practical initiatives being taken in the NHS to operationalise the MLCF and to provide new opportunities for doctors to gain managerial and leadership experiences and competences at earlier stages in their careers.

The MLCF has been designed to apply to all doctors in the numerous organisational and clinical settings in which they work. This means, therefore, that in future all medical students and postgraduate doctors will be required to attain the agreed set of leadership competences.

It is inevitable that there will be a differential pace of inclusion and indeed effectiveness in terms of impact. It would also be wrong to assume that management and leadership competences have not been hitherto incorporated into both undergraduate and postgraduate curricula and programmes. Many of the former incorporated some of the MLCF competences into professionalism standards, and most postgraduate deaneries and a number of colleges have offered management courses for specialist registrars. However, hitherto there has been no agreed set of consistent standards or competences to underpin the random offerings made available.

This chapter offers a sample of some interesting initiatives being taken within the medical educational and service environments. The sample is by no means exhaustive but demonstrates that the medical profession is rising to the challenge of equipping all doctors with the appropriate leadership skills to be effective and competent practitioners.

It is perhaps during postgraduate training that some of the best example of new programmes and other leadership development interventions are appearing. A number of them are described below, namely:

- Integrated Leadership Development throughout postgraduate training, London Specialty School of Paediatrics
- 'Prepare to Lead', a leadership development mentoring programme for specialist and GP registrars in London
- 'Lead or be Led', NHS Education South Central
- 'Stepping-Up to Your Leadership Role': the programme that facilitates your transition to consultant, University of Warwick Medical School
- Clinical Fellowships.

INTEGRATED LEADERSHIP DEVELOPMENT THROUGHOUT POSTGRADUATE TRAINING, LONDON SPECIALTY SCHOOL OF PAEDIATRICS

The London Specialty School of Paediatrics has piloted an approach to leadership development which, as Klaber stresses, 'integrates it throughout all years of training and embeds it within workplace-based learning' (Klaber, Roueché, Hodgkinson et al., 2008, p. 122). The programme acknowledges that, even if the principles of leadership are taught at an earlier stage in training, there need to be real opportunities for practising and developing them in a meaningful way.

Klaber et al. had difficulty in selecting the 30 trainees across all levels of training from the considerable number expressing interest in participating in the pilot programme; it is interesting to note that many more doctors are now expressing interest in the ever-increasing number of leadership development initiatives.

The 30 trainees were selected to be members of the training committee on the premise that after a day-and-a-half leadership development course, they would have ongoing opportunity to work in small groups alongside the training programme directors in one of seven key areas, i.e.:

- recruitment and workforce planning
- supporting trainees
- assessment of trainees
- curriculum development
- faculty development
- communications and IT
- research and audit.

During the initial day-and-a-half leadership course, participants were introduced to key concepts around medical leadership. This included undertaking a Myers-Briggs Type Indicator (MBTI) assessment, learning about some of the organisational structures within the NHS and to role-play a departmental meeting.

During the programme the participants generated ideas about how, as postgraduate trainees, they could develop their leadership skills during their day-to-day work.

The workplace opportunities to develop leadership skills as a postgraduate trainee developed by this group of junior doctors are listed in Box 9.1 below.

Box 9.1 Workplace opportunities to develop leadership skills as a postgraduate trainee

    Department induction

    Guideline development

    Rota management

    Identifying areas for change

    Teaching, education and supervision

    People management and performance management

    Attending and contributing to meetings

    Operational matters

    Service quality and improvements

    Identifying key players in the trust

    Understanding trust strategy

    National strategy

Source: Klaber *et al.*, 2008

'PREPARE TO LEAD': A LEADERSHIP DEVELOPMENT MENTORING PROGRAMME FOR SPECIALIST AND GP REGISTRARS IN LONDON

'Prepare to Lead' is a leadership development programme for specialist and general practitioner registrars working within the London Deanery and was launched in May 2008 with a second programme that started in April 2009. It has provoked considerable interest across the NHS, and many Strategic Health Authorities are implementing variations of the programme.

As Warren *et al.* (2008) confirm, 'Prepare to Lead' was established to respond to the strategic challenge articulated in Professor Darzi's report *A Framework for Action*, published in July 2007. This report suggested that NHS London needed to identify clinical champions to make the case for change to their public and that clinical leadership should be the key driver to making change and improvement happen.

'Prepare to Lead' attempts to equip selected participants with an understanding of the issues faced by NHS leaders and some of the essential skills required to take on significant leadership roles as they progress through their medical careers.

Over a 12-month period, the programme provides participants with mentoring from a senior healthcare leader and opportunities to shadow their mentor, work with him or her on small projects and attend various networking opportunities. Further learning opportunities are provided through a series of seminars, courses and workshops.

Warren reports that: 'feedback from the current group regarding uni-professional and multi-professional cohorts has been consistently in favour of uni-professional work' (Warren *et al.*, 2008).

Given that doctors inevitably work in multi-professional teams, this might seem strange, even more so as the Medical Leadership Competency Framework has now been adopted by all other clinical professions.

However, Warren *et al.* suggest that there are some specific reasons for this perspective, including that 'in contrast to many other healthcare professionals, moving into managerial and leadership roles is not regarded in many of their organisations as a natural career progression or something to which to aspire'.

They also noted that the lack of understanding of even basic issues, e.g. organisational arrangements, might be a barrier to multi-professional development at this stage. However, it is interesting that now this group have a good basic understanding, they would be keen to undertake further learning and development in multi-professional teams.

One of the great attributes of this particular programme is the 'duality' relationship between almost entirely non-medical mentors and medical mentees – not to mention the opportunity of shared learning and creating the value of this 'managerial:medical' duality relationship at an early stage for young doctors – a concept that the high-performing health organisations and systems in the USA possess at all levels.

LEAD OR BE LED: NHS EDUCATION SOUTH CENTRAL

Another example of the type of leadership development initiative being offered to and taken up by postgraduate trainee doctors is a two-day residential course offered by the Innovation and Development Courses Centre within NHS Education South Central.

As Livermore, a surgical trainee (Year 1) comments, 'Like most junior doctors I have spent a lot of time ranting about different NHS policies that affect me at a clinical level and how they do not seem to reflect the needs of patients or staff' (Livermore, 2010, p. GP16).

The programme is designed to meet the needs of junior doctors who hitherto have not received any formal teaching on leadership, teamwork or management either at medical school or during their postgraduate training.

This particular programme is multidisciplinary and includes specialist registrars, senior nurses and allied health professionals and trainee managers.

The content includes:

• key concepts around the structure and management of the NHS
• the Myers-Briggs personality instrument
• running an executive meeting
• presenting to a simulation of a government health select committee.

This simulation is run by a team of former chief executives, medical directors, journalists and politicians.

We agree with Livermore (2010), who concluded that such leadership development programmes should not be left too late in a doctor's training. Over the next few years we would anticipate that this type of programme and others described in this chapter will increasingly become the norm.

THE 'STEPPING-UP TO YOUR LEADERSHIP ROLE': the programme that facilitates your transition to consultant, University of Warwick Medical School

Another example of an innovative programme for postgraduate trainee doctors is the 'Stepping-Up' programme offered by the Institute for Clinical Leadership at the University of Warwick Medical School. Its aim is to prepare specialist registrars for the passage from trainee to clinical leader. The five-day programme is designed to equip trainees with the knowledge and skills to make the transition as smooth and effective as possible.

Based on the MLCF (NHS Institute for Innovation and Improvement, Academy of Medical Royal Colleges, 2010), it aims to:

- increase knowledge and understanding of the context and organisation of the health system
- explore the respective roles of the consultant in the health system and other medical management roles
- build confidence and self-insight into the effectiveness of personal leadership styles and behaviours and to link that to the performance of the 'consultant' role
- build confidence in working in the system, i.e. putting knowledge and skills into practice in different organisational situations such as negotiating resources and system improvement
- ensure an understanding of effective team-working in a multidisciplinary context.

The programme is delivered in two modules of two and three days. Participants are asked to undertake one small piece of preparatory work outlining a development project they would like to see for their particular specialty or service. This reinforces the authors' views that clinicians need to see the relevance of training in management and leadership as relevant to their roles as clinical practitioners.

The development proposal has to meet a range of criteria, including being:

- focused on a change, development or improvement related to the participant's specialty. The idea may require specific investment from the trust and/or one or more commissioner(s), and thought is required as to the likely scale of that investment and how it will be funded
- something that the participant is passionate about and would be prepared to implement
- clear about the benefits that would be realised by the change: to patients, to outcome, to reputation, to staff, to income and expenditure position. Particular consideration has to be given to quality, productivity and performance improvement

- clear about the impact of the idea on other specialties within the participant's organisation or other organisations in the health economy
- mindful of any potential risks inherent in implementing the change: clinical, financial, reputational or other.

CLINICAL FELLOWSHIPS

In Chapter 5 we referred to the development of 'Clinical Leadership Fellowships' within the NHS (England). Whilst given momentum by explicit reference in *High Quality Care for All* (Darzi, 2008), a number of earlier initiatives within, e.g. the chief medical officer's office and enlightened deaneries and trusts, had provided useful exemplars. London Strategic Health Authority and the London Deanery have led the way in which trusts (particularly acute hospitals) have offered a minimum of one clinical leadership fellow specifically to lead a clinical service improvement project across the local health economy within the trust. This programme is particularly open to specialist registrars and is designed to help develop the organisational and leadership skills necessary for their future roles as consultants, general practitioners and clinical leaders. The 'Darzi Clinical Leadership Fellows' are supported by a management and organisational change programme, including action learning and mentoring support. Participants also complete a postgraduate certificate 'Doctors as Managers' from Leeds University Business School.

These one-year fellowships are proving to be highly popular, with interest from specialist registrars considerably exceeding the number of opportunities. Equally, the interest from chief executives is refreshing and is perhaps a demonstration of the acknowledgement by non-medical executives of the value of securing greater engagement of doctors in leadership at a much earlier formative stage of their careers.

In general, the Darzi Fellowships are likely to comprise three elements outlined in Box 9.2 below:

Box 9.2 Key elements of the Darzi Fellowships

1. Change management project	Working with the medical director or another senior leader to support the development of service change ideally across organisational boundaries
2. Quality improvement/safety improvement/clinical governance project	Devising, leading and delivering a local quality and safety improvement and clinical governance initiative within the trust
3. Supporting capacity building within the trust for training in generic skills	Development of capacity for training in one or more of the essential organisational skills, e.g. teamworking, and to roll this out to specialist registrars (SpRs) and other clinical healthcare professionals

The former Chief Medical Officer's Clinical Advisory Scheme (CALS) has now been superceded by the Medical Director's Clinical Fellowship Programme. It provides opportunities to about 15 postgraduate trainee doctors to be seconded to a range of national and regional bodies for up to a year. Each doctor is mentored by a senior medical leader and is required to take on a challenging project as well as participate in a leadership development programme. This programme is now led by the newly established Faculty of Medical Leadership and Management.

Other strategic health authorities and deaneries are now following the example set by London and the Clinical Advisory and Clinical Fellowship Schemes. For example, the North West Deanery, in conjunction with the North West Leadership Academy, has also introduced an innovative leadership programme for specialist registrars. They not only undertake service improvement projects but also study for a postgraduate health leadership qualification and take on a number of development activities with trainees on the highly acclaimed NHS Graduate Management Training Scheme. This leadership capacity building programme has been in existence for over 50 years and many of today's chief executives (including four of the past five NHS Chief Executives in England) and other senior leaders are graduates of this scheme. It now recruits around 150 trainees each year in England; similar schemes exist in the other home countries.

The examples cited of recent leadership development initiatives for postgraduate trainees serve to reinforce how the medical profession is taking seriously the need for doctors to attain leadership competences early in their careers.

Whilst historically there have been similar ad hoc initiatives, the difference now is that the medical leadership movement is being embedded into a doctors training and experience supported by all the medical professional, regulatory and educational bodies. Similarly, NHS organisations are increasingly recognising their responsibility to provide such leadership development opportunities.

However, it would be wrong to suggest that identifying specific leadership project roles for specialist registrars is revolutionary. Historically, a number of ad hoc posts have been created to lead specific medical initiatives, e.g. implementation of the European Working Time Directive (EWTD). What appears to be different this time is that there is a sustained movement to create organisational cultures that positively encourage doctors to take time out from their specialist clinical training to develop leadership and project management skills. The attitude of deaneries has also changed from one where any distraction from the specialist training programme was generally frowned upon to increasingly one where positive encouragement is offered.

CONTINUING PRACTICE

Whilst there have been an increasing number of new leadership development opportunities particularly for postgraduate trainee doctors, many trusts are recognising the importance of developing in-house leadership programmes for newly appointed consultants and general practitioners. Some of the early evidence from those organisations with high levels of engagement of doctors in management, leadership and transformation of services – and corresponding high performance – is the importance they attach to such in-house development programmes.

Some of these in-house programmes are uni-disciplinary; others multi-professional. Some follow the MLCF as the underpinning model to inform the content of the programme, and others focus on the key strategic issues of the trust. The important point is that trusts are increasingly recognising the value of engaging newly appointed doctors with their strategic plans and modus operandi.

In addition to in-house programmes for newly appointed specialists, some deaneries are also providing leadership development opportunities. A number of these initiatives are described below, namely:

- introduction to leadership and management for GPs
- intensive induction for consultants: 'a signature experience'
- 'Fit to Lead'.

INTRODUCTION TO LEADERSHIP AND MANAGEMENT FOR GPS

Another example of opportunities for management and leadership development for any GP who has graduated from the Vocational Training Scheme within the last five years is offered by the Institute of Clinical Leadership at the University of Warwick Medical School.

The course is offered over four afternoons and evenings and one full day, and it provides opportunities to develop management and leadership skills based around the MLCF. It includes self-assessment, multi-source feedback, structure and function of the NHS, finance, employment, team-working, networking and negotiation, practice-based commissioning, project management, business planning, how to run a PCT, CV writing and career planning.

Again, this programme includes a project linked to the participants' roles in primary care with an emphasis on relevance and capability for implementation.

INTENSIVE INDUCTION FOR CONSULTANTS: A 'SIGNATURE EXPERIENCE'

It is evident that traditionally most consultants and general practitioners have had little, if any, formal leadership development prior to taking up such important and influential roles. With the mandatory nature of the MLCF, this should change for the next generation. However, many trusts are recognising the importance of providing an intensive induction for newly appointed consultants and general practitioners. One example of this is at Barnsley PCT NHS Trust.

Chari and Rele (2008) argue that 'there is little doubt that for those in hospital practice, becoming a consultant is important, and if not a pinnacle of achievement, is at least a stop-over on the way to such levels of achievement' (p. 89).

They also confirm that the 'transition from specialist registrar to consultant is a challenging but important journey adding that "a feeling of being thrown in at the deep end" is not uncommon, and causes anxiety. During the initial years of specialist training, the emphasis is on improving one's clinical skills and taking responsibility. There is little emphasis on key management issues' (p. 89).

As a consequence, an intensive induction process has been developed for a number of newly appointed consultants. This includes a number of regular sessions with the medical director, mandatory corporate induction and one-to-one meetings with members of senior management, including the chairman, chief executive and other executive directors.

The particular example from Barnsley PCT NHS Trust is not unique. A number of other trusts, including most of those with the highest medical engagement scale index (*see* Chapter 7) have also recognised the importance of valuing new consultants and general practitioners and securing their commitment to the trust and local community served.

Given the wide range of extra-clinical demands and opportunities for consultants and general practitioners and the ever-increasing need for clinicians to be business and quality-focused, trusts need to be alert to every opportunity to secure the engagement of key and potentially long-serving staff.

THE BRITISH ASSOCIATION OF MEDICAL MANAGERS: 'FIT TO LEAD'

The British Association of Medical Managers (BAMM) had a long tradition of offering management and leadership development support to medical managers, i.e. those in positional leadership roles. Established in 1991, BAMM was an independent registered charity and provided a strong national voice for the importance of medical management over the past two decades before its demise in 2010.

BAMM developed its own 'Fit to Lead' programme. This set a structure and framework for medical leadership and management. It was based on a framework of Standards of Medical Management and Leadership developed in conjunction with a wide range of medical leaders at all levels of the NHS and across all disciplines.

'Fit to Lead' measured the knowledge and skills already in place and, through a tutoring process, identified a personal development programme. As part of the programme, BAMM included a three-day 'Skills Factory' based around the Standards of Medical Leadership and Management. It was a certified programme and offered three attainment levels:

- Certified Medical Manager (CMM)
- Advanced Medical Leader (AML)
- BAMM Fellow.

Other providers are now offering their own development programmes for those in, or preparing for, positional medical leadership roles. These include short courses for clinical and medical directors either in-house or through an increasing range of providers.

POSTGRADUATE LEADERSHIP DEGREES, UNIVERSITY OF WARWICK

Historically, few doctors whether in practitioner or leadership roles have undertaken postgraduate degrees in, for example, business administration, health policy and leadership. A number of universities are now offering tailored master's in Medical Leadership.

The University of Warwick commenced an MSc in Medical Leadership in 2008. Led by the Medical School, the programme is delivered in conjunction with the Clinical Systems Improvement Unit and Business School. Thirty consultants and general practitioners are participating in the initial two-year, part-time master's programme covering the following core modules:

- Leadership for Doctors
- NHS Strategy, Policy and Organisation
- Systems Approach to Patient Safety
- Clinical Systems Improvement
- Comparative Health Care Systems.

In addition to studying other optional modules, the students are required to undertake a professional project or dissertation. During the Comparative Health Care Systems module, the students get an opportunity to join similar master's students at another university, e.g. Erasmus in Rotterdam. This provides a great opportunity to reflect on the way in which healthcare is organised and delivered in the NHS with a different system.

As previous chapters have confirmed, the NHS has embarked on a service and quality improvement journey that requires more doctors to take the lead in driving change. It is evident that leadership development initiatives that embrace the service improvement movement are far more likely to be attractive to doctors than those that historically were more focused around resource and business management.

INNOVATIVE DEVELOPMENT INITIATIVES

It would be wrong to suggest that all leadership development initiatives have emanated within deaneries, strategic health authorities and other national bodies.

The following boxes offer a number of examples of good practice that demonstrate the variety of approaches that individuals and organisations are adopting:

What these examples demonstrate is that there is a wide range of ways in which doctors during their postgraduate training can contribute to service improvement. In addition, they demonstrate that securing greater medical engagement depends not only on doctors wanting to widen their contribution but also on other more senior doctors and leaders creating such opportunities.

Box 9.3 Some examples of innovative development initiatives

On the first day of joining the healthcare organisation, Foundation Year (FY) 1 doctors met, as a group, with the trust medical director. At that meeting, the medical director asked the FY1 doctors to record every time they saw a service issue that resulted in patients receiving suboptimal care. A few weeks later, when the FY1 doctors met again with the medical director, they were asked what issues they had recorded and what they had done to correct or improve the service issue for patients. This simple action by the medical director emphasised that it was the responsibility of all doctors to improve services for patients and empowered junior doctors to be involved.

***

When David was an SpR, the chief executive of the organisation in which he worked regularly met with SpRs informally and used them as a temperature check for how the organisation was performing.

The chief executive also involved SpRs as part of the consultant group following a public enquiry into patient care. SpRs were invited to many meetings where sensitive and difficult issues about the organisation were discussed.

By doing this, the chief executive demonstrated good leadership and a keen interest in the doctors and the service. This was unlike any previous experience David had had of a medical manager or board member. Such a positive example encouraged David to become involved in medical management and leadership.

***

As a junior doctor, Susan became interested in service improvement. Her desire to improve the service and system in which she worked led her to seek a dual role as service modernisation lead and trust specialist.

Susan was encouraged to establish this role by a number of senior leaders in her hospital who helped her develop a business case for the new role, which was approved by the trust board.

Susan now devotes half her time as a trust specialist in general internal medicine and the remaining half on service improvement projects such as redesigning emergency access and medical pathways.

In her service improvement role, Susan has found that she has an advantage of having worked in most clinical departments and therefore has a good understanding of the procedures and issues faced by each department.

***

An SHA and two deaneries took a unique and innovative approach to achieving compliance with the EWTD. Six junior doctor advisors led by a junior doctor manager were recruited for a team that was responsible for ensuring full directive compliance was achieved for all junior doctors in training by August 2008.

Junior doctors in the team drew upon their knowledge and experience to provide expert, impartial advice while providing a performance management role to ensure all trusts comply with the EWTD. They influenced changes to working practices and rota planning.

The position provided these junior doctors with a wealth of managerial experience and helped them develop skills such as negotiation, communication, presentation, budgeting and line management. These doctors have developed a greater understanding of management roles and pressures and gained experience that will be useful throughout their careers.

***

A dentist specialising in maxillofacial surgery noticed a high cancellation and delay rate in transplant operations for children. The delays occurred due to problems with getting children's teeth checked before the transplant.

There was no system in place, with the children just fitted into already crowded clinics. The delays caused not only great distress to the children and families but also great problems with the rest of the team dealing with these very sick children.

The dentist was able to update the care pathway, working with the transplant coordinator to ensure there was designated clinic time for children in her routine work, ensuring timely examination.

She also worked with the general dental practitioners in primary care for appropriate checks to be done in a community setting; ensuring problems would be seen as part of the routine outpatient work.

No clinic felt overstretched by extra work, the coordinators knew when the children were going to be seen and the families were able to experience a seamless and trouble-free pathway prior to the transplant.

***

A GP chose to work in an inner-city practice because of his interest in diabetes. Within a few months he noticed an ongoing delay in initiating insulin for patients who had type 2 diabetes. Upon investigation, he found these delays were caused by a very long wait to see the dietician, before a longer wait to be seen in the classes run by the diabetes specialist nurses.

He worked with the practice manager and made a business case for the practice to employ a dietician for a session a week, then found a training course for himself, one of the other doctors, a practice nurse and a district nurse to attend, enabling them to initiate insulin in house.

Further work with the primary care trust (PCT) attracted a locally enhanced service payment, which offset the extra time spent with the patients. The dietician was also able to see patients with other health issues, and more patients were seen and treated in the community. The PCT used this scheme to design a care pathway for other practices to do the same thing.

There are a range of e-learning packages to help doctors learn about leadership and management. LeAD is a free and engaging e-learning resource to help doctors develop their understanding of how their role contributes to managing and leading health services. LeAD comprises over 50 sessions of highly interactive e-learning in support of the MLCF.

MEDICAL AND CLINICAL LEADERSHIP DEVELOPMENT?

The term 'clinical leadership' is all too often used when meaning 'medical leadership'. However, the arguments used to support the importance of doctors acquiring leadership competences in order to be good doctors equally apply to all other clinical professionals. *High Quality Care for All* (Darzi, 2008) recognised the need to increase the supply of high-quality leadership within the NHS and identified that there were not enough clinical professionals willing and able to take on leadership roles.

Work is now underway to extend the MLCF to all clinical professionals as part of a new standard for healthcare leadership with certification at a number of levels ranging from the MLCP (as revised for all clinical professionals) as the initial level and chief executive or equivalent as the highest level.

This initiative is part of the new NHS National Leadership Council vision of creating an NHS with outstanding leadership and leadership development at every level. Given the strong governmental emphasis on the importance of clinical leadership and engagement, it is not surprising that one of the key priority areas is clinical leadership and removing the barriers to enable more leadership positions to be filled by clinicians.

It will be interesting to observe over the next decade whether the focus and investment in clinical (and particularly medical) leadership impacts on the professional background of senior leaders in the NHS.

Earlier we referred to the NHS Graduate Management Training Scheme (MTS) as being a major pipeline for the current cadre of chief executives and directors. From recruiting about 15 trainees back in 1956, it has now grown to a scheme whereby around 200 are recruited each year across the NHS (UK). The 'fast-track' programme offers a range of development opportunities including working attachments, action learning, mentoring, post-graduate studies and regular performance review. Hitherto, most of the development, with a few variations, is undertaken as a uni-disciplinary group within the multi-professional culture of NHS organisations and services.

A rethink of the overall approach to preparing clinical and non-clinical staff for their managerial and leadership roles is emerging. One or two opportunities have been taken over the past few years to create joint learning, but this now needs to become more systematic. This includes an initiative to create 'buddying' relationships between each management trainee and a junior doctor. This creates early opportunities for young managers and clinicians to recognise the value of working and developing together as dualities.

We believe that we shall see more senior leaders from clinical backgrounds in the future, as a result of the various policy and local initiatives and investments encouraging greater engagement and offering leadership development at all levels of a doctor's training.

What is unclear is whether this will improve the quality and productivity of the NHS. Whilst as Chapter 7 has demonstrated, securing greater engagement of doctors in the planning, delivery and transformation of services does have an impact on quality and efficiency, there is no evidence whatsoever that medical leaders are more effective than non-medical leaders. Hitherto, there have not been sufficient numbers to undertake a proper evaluation.

These experiences and the changing nature of the NHS agenda, with such a strengthened focus on service improvement – including quality and safety and new professional paradigms – suggest that a new multi-professional approach to the development of managers and leaders is required.

The Future of Leadership and Management in the NHS: no more heroes (2011) stresses that every NHS organisation and provider must take responsibility for leadership and management development. This includes the new GP Consortia. The report from The Kings Fund suggests that one of the biggest weaknesses of the NHS has been its failure to engage doctors in a sustained way in management and leadership. However, the report rightly argues that 'development in both leadership and management is needed for a much wider range of staff than just doctors' (2011, p. 21). As this chapter has demonstrated, leadership development should focus not only on technical competencies but also on service improvement. The past reluctance of clinicians to take leadership development seriously, particularly where focussed on resource management, appears to be changing rapidly with the new attention on service improvement.

REFERENCES

Chari S, Rele K. Intensive induction for consultants: a 'signature experience'. *The International Journal of Clinical Leadership*. 2008; **16**(2): 89–95.

Darzi A. *Healthcare for London: a framework for action*. London: NHS London; 2007.

Darzi A. *High Quality Care for All: NHS Next Stage Review Final Report*. London: Department of Health; 2008.

Klaber RE, Roueché A, Hodgkinson R, *et al*. A structured approach to planning a work-based leadership development programme for doctors in training. *The International Journal of Clinical Leadership*. 2008; **16**(3): 121–9.

Livermore LJ. Lead or be led. *BMJ Careers*. 2010; **340**: 59–108.

NHS Institute for Innovation and Improvement, Academy of Medical Royal Colleges. *Medical Leadership Competency Framework*. 3rd ed. Coventry: NHS Institute for Innovation and Improvement; 2010.

The King's Fund. *The Future of Leadership and Management in the NHS: no more heroes*. London: The King's Fund; 2011.

Warren OJ, Humphris P, Bicknell CD. 'Prepare to Lead': reflections on the first year of a leadership programme for specialist and GP registrars in London. *The International Journal of Clinical Leadership*. 2008; **16**(3): 149–55.

CHAPTER 10

Medical leadership: towards cultural acceptance and the future

Previous chapters have given an account of widespread recognition and evidence of the need for greater engagement of doctors in the management and leadership tasks that support the achievement of improved healthcare delivery. Each health system has its own history and process of evolution, but there appears to be consensus about the requirement for the powerful profession of medicine to be positively integrated into both strategic and operational aspects of running health services.

Mountford (2010) argues that the time has come for clinical leadership to emerge as a significant factor in the way health services are run. He cites issues such as the complexity of policy changes, the safety and quality imperative and the gradually emerging evidence of the impact of clinical leadership on organisational performance. Similarly, Bohmer (2010) calls for leadership training, both high-level system leadership and more leadership with an operational focus, to be built into the training and preparation of all doctors.

In many ways there would seem to be little of a radical or startling nature in advocating such a role for doctors. In many systems, especially in earlier versions of healthcare structures, doctors have always played a prominent role and still do in many current systems (*see* Chapter 5). However, there are two particular contextual issues that seem to make the notion of enhanced medical leadership quite challenging.

The first concerns the peculiar nature of the personal services provided by doctors. In many other sectors the key professions have had less difficulty integrating their role within the constraints of a managed system. For example, architects, engineers and designers – despite their frustrations – will recognise the interactive dynamic (and constraints) of the system in which they work. Many groups of this type work in a collective system, whereas doctors are largely delivering a highly personalised, individually based service. It can also of course be a highly emotive service where quality of life, as well as life or death, may be involved. Doctors and the public, as patients, have something akin to an implicit contract that the individual transaction around care giving shall remain the predominant characteristic of health systems. Anything externally imposed that impinges upon this relationship tends to be resented, and this perspective has been how many doctors have viewed managers and management.

A critical cultural challenge for the future is to overcome this quite widely held view and build an approach that recognises the wider system context but without detriment to the crucial patient-doctor relationship.

A second and related issue is that of clinical autonomy. Politicians in many systems have quite legitimate concerns about the escalating cost of healthcare and also more latterly around patient safety. These concerns have frequently manifested themselves as centralised interventions to reduce or control spending or to insist on certain forms of care delivery. Inevitably many doctors have seen such initiatives as constraining the way they work and thereby affecting their clinical autonomy to practice in accord with their professional values. It is argued that this increasingly centralised approach has created a somewhat alienated medical workforce and that the momentum towards forms of medical leadership is recognition of the need to alter this perspective. The *NHS Next Stage Review* as presented by Lord Darzi (2008) was an attempt to be more receptive and consultative towards the medical profession, and to refocus attention on quality and patient safety as issues more likely to be embraced by doctors in improving care overall. There is no doubt that this approach has contributed significantly to the impetus to see enhanced engagement in medical leadership. A new coalition government in the UK has continued to reinforce the need to put clinicians at the forefront of key decisions. As health systems move into the severe constraints of post-recession economies, it is imperative that this positive focus is maintained. Radical change and leading edge innovation in how services are provided will be fundamental to coping with the financial pressures. These will not be achieved without the full and positive engagement of medical staff (and others of course). Medical leadership in this climate is not an optional extra or a nicety but an essential ingredient.

MISCONCEPTIONS ABOUT MANAGEMENT AND LEADERSHIP

As outlined earlier in this text, there are many models of leadership, many misconceptions about the nature and purpose of management and many unhelpful stereotypes. If medical leadership, as advocated here, is to flourish and become a normal and accepted component of the medical career, then these stereotypes need to be challenged and reframed into a more modern 21st century way of thinking.

In advocating that all doctors should acquire competence in management and leadership and that these functions are integral to the professional role, there is no suggestion that doctors should become managers rather than doctors or that each doctor is naturally (by selection into medical school) equipped to be a heroic or charismatic positional leader. Managerial tasks are essential to the effective operation of large organisations. The majority of these will continue to be undertaken by managers, but doctors by developing a better understanding of the function and purpose of these tasks can contribute significantly to their functional effectiveness. The management process can no longer be seen as an alien and – as described by some – deliberately undermining to good healthcare delivery. There can of course be poor managers and poor examples of management. Systems can become perseverated and unwieldy, but to regard all management as hostile and deficient is to perpetuate a cultural divide that is not only unhelpful but unreasonable.

Similarly, to embrace medical leadership in such a way as to suggest that doctors must be the dominant players in an explicitly multi-professional, team-based delivery system is inappropriate and outmoded. The model of shared or distributed leadership as described in Chapter 3 is much more the type of leadership that is needed in the complex health systems of today. Such a model of leadership is essentially flexible, recognising the expertise and contribution of others as and when appropriate, empowering such as to release the skills of others to improve overall performance, and consultative in attempting to ensure that the ideas and abilities of others are brought into play. This is a long way from the dominant dictatorial stereotype of the authoritarian leader of the past.

Lee (2010) reinforces this view, suggesting that a new breed of medical leaders is required to meet the challenges of providing 21st century healthcare. He particularly emphasises the development of teams as a key leadership strategy for healthcare providers. He cites the experience of Geisinger Health System in Pennsylvania, where such arrangements have helped the hospital cut re-admission rates by half. Lee suggests that a critical component of this success is 'that physicians be both team leaders and team players' (p. 57). Building teams and inspiring teamwork comprise an important competence for leaders in order to improve performance.

Just as we talk of enhancing engagement in medical leadership so we need to develop engaging leaders able to relate, empathise and influence others, to build teams that are clear about their roles and motivated to perform them and with the intellectual flexibility to adapt to often fluctuating and contradictory demands.

THE FUTURE OF MEDICAL LEADERSHIP

On a number of occasions within this text, the nature and picture of medical leadership described has been represented as a significant cultural change. It requires that medical leadership skills are embedded into medical training and medical career development as an important and established element of professionalism. The Medical Leadership Competency Framework (*see* Chapter 8) is perhaps the most important recent initiative in this respect for decades. Its incorporation into the training of undergraduate medical students will lead to an awareness and understanding of how these skills are relevant to future roles in medicine as well as beginning the process of acquiring competence in them. Further development at the postgraduate level should ensure doctors are much more competent in the demands of system management, improvement methodologies and leadership; it should also ensure they emerge with a more positive attitude to the contribution they can make to the management process.

In the UK, at least this process of development and acquisition of competence in management and leadership may continue further into the period of continuing practice following specialist certification. This is dependent upon current consultation around the forthcoming processes of medical revalidation. The process of revalidation will be overseen by the General Medical Council (GMC) and will be aimed at assuring patients, the public and employers that doctors are up to date and fit to practice. Revalidation will be based around the annual appraisal, which will involve evaluation of the doctor's performance against professional standards set by the GMC and the Medical Royal Colleges. *Good Medical Practice* is the document produced by the GMC, and this defines the standards of care required, and a set of standards framework for appraisal and assessment has been devised. Inclusion or cross-referencing of these standards to the Medical Leadership Competency Framework would therefore ensure that practising doctors continue to refine and develop their leadership skills alongside their clinical work.

These changes to preparation and the attitude of doctors to management and leadership will not happen overnight, hence the notion of cultural change. But the hostile, unproductive divide between managers and doctors will hopefully be replaced by a more positive recognition and respect for a complementary set of skills. In order for this to happen the roles taken by doctors (and hence role models) as clinical leads, clinical directors, medical directors and the like must be accepted and valued as a normal component of the medical career. If they are to become valued in this way, it will be important that the reward systems are aligned such that there is no disincentive for doctors to play a full role in the management and leadership of their organisation. Already junior doctor rotations are beginning to include management and leadership placements that would once have been viewed as unthinkable. The authors have recently interviewed all current NHS chief executives with a medical background in order to identify how those who make this transition may be assisted in the process. (Ham, Clark, Spurgeon, 2010). It is not the goal of supporters of medical leadership to see all chief executives as medical in background. However, the current under-representation (23 out of approximately 350 positions) does suggest a lack of attraction to such roles. A better balance with more competent doctors – trained and equipped in management and leadership – working alongside high-level managers would surely be good for the health service.

The difficulties that were encountered by doctors moving into chief executive roles (Ham, Clark, Spurgeon, 2010) are very similar to the experiences of those taking on medical leadership roles. If the cultural change sought (in other words, a positive valuing and attraction to these roles) is to be achieved, then a number of key facilitators will need to be put in place. These include, for example:

- clearer career paths that provide opportunities for doctors to experience different leadership roles and to be offered appropriate development (coaching, learning sets) to move into them
- the reviewal of pay and reward systems so that medical leadership roles are properly recognised
- the facilitation of re-training if necessary so that the choice to move towards a leadership role is not seen as final and irrevocable.

A clear message from the study of medically qualified chief executives was that 'the time has come to adopt a more structured and systematic approach to medical leadership in the NHS' (p. 5). As part of this process, an important recent step has seen the establishment of a Faculty of Medical Leadership. This will provide a focus of professional identity for those individuals moving into these hybrid medical/leadership roles. It will also conduct research and advise as to best practice in developing leadership skills and ensure high standards across the entire workforce, from undergraduate level to national leaders, in the provision of training and development.

It is interesting to note that a number of chief executive appointments in the last six months have been made from candidates with a medical background. The growth of medical leadership is of its time, a cultural zeitgeist focusing healthcare delivery on quality and safety, and radical change and improvement. Earlier chapters have traced the history of this process, including a number of barriers and difficulties en route. An account has also been provided of key initiatives and changes in attitude that will inevitably see a sustained growth in medical leaders – both more competent in the requisite skill set and positively engaged with the wider goals of healthcare organisations and the demands of society upon medical professionals in the 21st century.

Some recently published work in Australia by Kippist and Fitzgerald (2009) provides a helpful tailpiece to what may be seen as the underpinning rationale to this text and many of the initiatives described within it. The authors explore the well-documented tensions inherent in the hybrid role of clinician manager, notably the potential conflict between clinical priorities and managerial goals. Apart from the pressures on time and lack of clarity of role, they point to a significant potential inhibitor to the success of such hybrid roles, namely the lack of management expertise held by doctors suddenly thrust into making significant managerially based decisions. They rightly highlight the danger to the organisation of less well-qualified (managerially) individuals making managerial decisions. They cite a number of authors who have also documented aspects of this deficiency, for example, lack of awareness of the roles of other staff in the organisation (Ormrod, 1993), poor communication with fellow team members (Lopopolo et al., 2004) and less management training (Fitzgerald, 2002).

These pressures are fully recognised (*see* Chapter 3), but it is important to also recognise the particular cultural context (Australia) in terms of the place and status of medical leadership within the health system. Moreover, as the authors suggest, a critical missing ingredient in the successful adoption of medical leadership roles is for doctors to have had the necessary training and development in appropriate skills. The development and widespread adoption of the Medical Leadership Competency Framework into all levels of training and career development of doctors, as described and advocated here, would go a long way to off-setting the expertise deficiency and acceptability of the medical leadership role. As a final comment to this text, our ambition is to see medical professionalism incorporate the concepts of management and leadership, and to see both individuals and the medical profession embrace the potential of doctors to contribute to the wider goals of the organisation as a normal and natural part of the medical role.

REFERENCES

Bohmer R. Leadership with a small 'l'. *BMJ.* 2010; **340**: 265.

Darzi A. *High Quality Care for All: NHS Next Stage Review Final Report.* London: Department of Health; 2008.

Fitzgerald JA. *Doctors and Nurses Working Together: a mixed methodology in the construction of changing professional identifies.* Sydney, Australia: University of Western Sydney; 2002.

Ham C, Clark J, Spurgeon P, *et al. Medical Chief Executives in the NHS: facilitators and barriers to progress.* Coventry: NHS Institute for Innovation and Improvement, University of Warwick; 2010.

Kippist L, Fitzgerald A. Organisational professional conflict and hybrid clinician managers. *J Health Organ Manag.* 2009; **23**(6): 642–55.

Lee TH. Turning doctors into leaders. *Harvard Business Review.* 2010 April: 51–8.

Lopopolo RB, Schafer SD, Nosse LJ. Leadership, administration, management and professionalism (LAMP) in physical therapy: a Delphi study. *Phys Ther.* 2004; **84**(2):137–50.

Mountford J. Clinical leadership: bringing the strands together. In: Stanton E, Lemer C, Mountford J, editors. *Clinical Leadership: bridging the divide.* London: MA Healthcare; 2010.

Ormrod J. Decision making in health service managers. *Management Decision.* 1993; **31**(7): 8–14.

Index

Diagrams are given in italics.